PRAISE FOR REFUSE TO DIET:

"In *Refuse To Diet* Laurie Tossy is sharing with you the secret of weight loss and weight control. This is an extraordinary book capable of changing anyone's life. Thank you for giving the world such an incredible tool to finding the health within each of us."

~from the Foreward by Dr. Linda Larson
Your Health and Fitness Source

"As a person who's lost weight, regained weight and lost weight again, I found inspiration, encouragement and common sense in Laurie Tossy's book, *Refuse to Diet: Weight Loss Success Starts with Your Mind Not Your Mouth*.

Laurie reveals the truth about why a country obsessed with dieting is so overweight. If you want to reach your ideal weight, everything you need to know is hidden in plain sight between the pages of Laurie's book. But be warned...if you start applying these concepts, not only will you reach your ideal weight; your whole attitude about everything from money to relationships is likely to change as well. Laurie eloquently reminds us that changing our minds can change our bodies and our reality.

If you want to reclaim your personal power and step into the joy of your own authenticity, don't miss out on this book. Laurie writes with clarity, wit and keen observations that anyone (even skinny people!) will enjoy."

~Donna Kozik
2-Time Award Winning Author,
Founder of MyBigBusinessCard.com,
& the "Write a Book in a Weekend Club" on Facebook

"Laurie Tossy has hit a homerun with her new book *Refuse to Diet*, where she outlines a simply revolutionary approach to finally breaking the shackles of yo-yo dieting. The Mind has the power to propel us towards a goal or repel from one. Read *Refuse to Diet* and discover the key strategy to transforming your body and life forever."

~Andrew Skelly
Author, *The Amazing Millionaire Formula*

"*Refuse To Diet* is truly the BEST health and wellness book (or non-diet book) that I have ever read! This book provides information and motivation for readers to finally take control of their lives and successfully explains why changing our mindset has got to be the very first step in our process for successfully and permanently losing weight. Laurie provides easy to understand tips and tools that will guide and assist you towards reclaiming your personal power by exposing the obstacles and barriers that keep you stuck in repeating the same patterns over and over again. These tools will help you discover a new sense of vitality, confidence and sheer pleasure of being alive. This is a permanent solution for breaking the diet habit and gaining a healthy and energetic body for mental, emotional and physical wellness."

~Gena Livings
Personal Health and Fitness Coach

"I just finished reading your book, *Refuse to Diet*. In fact, I read it twice. This could revolutionize the way in which people approach weight loss. Congratulations on writing such a fine piece of work. This will be a life-changing book for a great many people."

~Ron Matthews
Certified Energy Medicine Practitioner

MORE FROM LAURIE TOSSY:

"Seven Secrets to Successful Weight Loss without Dieting," http://www.SuccessfulWeightLossWithoutDieting.com

Laurie's blog: http://refusetodiet.blogspot.com/

Laurie on Twitter: https://twitter.com/Laurie_Tossy

Laurie on Facebook: http://www.facebook.com/home.php?#/laurie.tossy

To learn more about Laurie and her system for achieving health and dropping fat visit her website at http://www.RefuseToDiet.com. There you can join a supportive community of people who are all pulling together to achieve their health goals, get weight loss tips and specific tools that you can use on a daily basis that actually work.

Refuse to Diet

Weight Loss Success Starts with Your Mind... Not Your Mouth

Laurie Tossy

Refuse to Diet

Weight Loss Success Starts with Your Mind...Not Your Mouth

ISBN: 978-0-9826193-0-8

Laurie Tossy
Paid To Empower, LLC
1151 Eagle Dr. Suite 144
Loveland, Colorado 80537
1-800-662-1961 x2784
Laurie@RefuseToDiet.com
http://www.RefuseToDiet.com

Author photos by Mike Tossy

Illustrations by the author

Limits of Liability and Disclaimer of Warranty

Material Connection Disclosure

Dedication

This book is dedicated to my partner, Cathy, for accepting me the way I was and am now. No matter my size and health, Cathy has always been my biggest supporter. Without her encouragement and prodding I wouldn't have actually gotten this book written. I am filled with gratitude for having someone in my life who saw past my weight and helped me to heal my spirit and my body.

Acknowledgements

I want to thank several people for helping me on my journey to health and for getting this book written.

Dr. Linda Larson is a good friend and my health coach, she really helped me to believe enough in myself to have success.
Dr. Linda has also been a fantastic support answering questions about health and nutrition so I have confidence that my results are permanent and positive for my overall health.

Dr. John Gray, who helped me to realize that while I was responsible for my choices, the food I ate impacted my ability to make good choices. His focus on gaining health as opposed to weight loss, and for shining a light on some of the lies I had been telling myself about weight loss, dieting and exercise.

Brent Payne was the person who said "success-failure: choose." He stressed that everything really is that simple: a choice. That started me to actually believe that I could choose health. This simple statement was the catalyst for the first step on my path to health and weight loss.

Donna Kozik for helping me to actually get this book written. Her guidance, support, and gentle kicks were essential in finally getting the words in print.

Mike Tossy, my brother, for taking my "after" photos.

And to every one of you who reads this book. I am aware of your struggles and am so looking forward to your triumphs!

Preface

Women have been told time and time again that it is important to be thin and at the same time that it is actually difficult to be thin. We are given the messages that either we will never succeed at losing weight because of our genes or that we are a failure because we have not succeeded. Somehow some of us manage to get and believe both those messages at the same time!

How many times have you gone on a diet with the best of intentions, starting off like a house-a-fire only to hit a stumbling block where you ended up eating something not on your diet? Not only did you lose momentum, but if you are like most people, it took you off the path entirely and you ended up gaining more weight than you had lost in the beginning. This leads to us beating ourselves up because we have these unrealistic standards.

What I do is show women who are frustrated with yo-yo dieting, who are tired of feeling bad about themselves, how to gain their health once and for all—without dieting!

I can do this because I have been there. In my life I have tried just about every diet there was, starting at eleven years of age. Just a few short years ago I was over 300 pounds, tired all the time, unhappy, on anti-depressants and prescription medication to control heart palpitations. I was told I would be on these medications the rest of my life. I didn't like that idea, but I had resigned myself to it. It wasn't until I decided to shift my mindset, and "unresign" myself that things began to change.

I have since lost over 125 pounds, gained energy and overall health and I am off all medications. I have been able to take control of my life and no longer suffer from cravings. What I have discovered is that pretty much everything we have been taught about dieting is a big fat lie! It is truly possible for everyone to achieve their ideal weight without having to be a slave at the gym or give up your favorite foods forever.

Not only do you not have to give up your favorite foods, you don't have to count calories or fat grams or go on any restrictive diet to achieve your health goals. There is no weighing food portions and no carrots instead of cookies—no deprivation.

Sound good? I will tell you, it is great! What made the difference? How is this possible, when all the "experts" tell you otherwise? I learned the key was about what was going on in my mind much more than what I put in my mouth.

If you have ever struggled with your weight, and if you aren't even sure that it is really possible to lose weight for good, then this book is for you. I'll share my story with you and show you how you, too, can start your own journey to regain your healthy body.

Foreward

We've all seen literally thousands of diets and weight loss plans. In January of every year the hype begins about some new diet, weight loss pill or exercise program that will make you slim like a model. NOT! The truth of the matter is that there is no magic diet, weight loss pill or exercise program. There is no fountain of youth.

The biggest health epidemic in this country at present is not cancer or heart disease, it is obesity. If you don't believe me, look around you. As a society we are getting fatter and fatter which is causing more illnesses and has resulted in an astronomical number of people becoming Diabetic. I know many of you have tried and maybe been successful in losing weight, only to put it back on plus more.

In this book, *Refuse To Diet* Laurie Tossy is sharing with you the secret of weight loss and weight control. I have watched Laurie struggle for years with her weight and try every formula out there in hopes of getting it under control. The secret is not some special pill, diet, or exercise program. The secret is within you and that is what she is sharing in this book.

Laurie gives you tools to begin to uncover the secret within you so that weight loss is no longer an effort where you feel deprived. That starts with understanding that your body may never have been designed to be the model's body and that is perfectly fine. Laurie gives you tips on how to accept and be OK with the body you have.

In helping Laurie in her process, I found that I too was learning about foods and what is good for us. I learned about the energy within the body and how to not only tap into that energy, but increase my energy through particular exercises which didn't require going to a gym or having a lot of equipment in my home. Laurie has given me some secrets that I can not only use in my own life, but also share with others who are struggling with their weight.

Laurie wrote this book for the average person who is struggling or has been struggling for years to lose weight. *Refuse To Diet* contains the tools for you to succeed in being the best you.

Laurie has learned from experience. If there is a diet out there she has tried it. She has also tried multiple "diet pills" which have not worked either. She has studied and worked with people who are experts in the fields of nutrition, exercise, and personal development. The hardest work she did was on her own personal development with the masters in this field. This is where Laurie learned that the secret was within her. She lived this experience and her sharing it with the world is an incredible gifts.

This is an extraordinary book capable of changing anyone's life and certainly their weight if they are willing to dig down deep and follow Laurie's lead. It's not about deprivation.

Thank you for giving the world such an incredible tool to finding the health within each of us. This is a great read containing many very useful tools.

Dr. Linda Larson

Your Health and Fitness Source

Table of Contents

Introduction

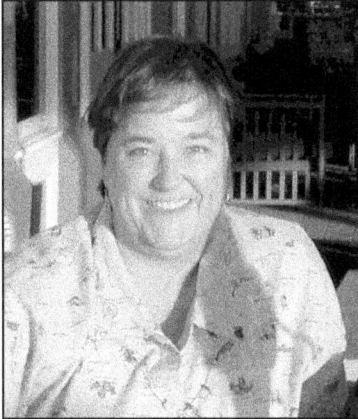

Would you take weight loss advice from this person? Probably not, but I did and am I ever glad. You see, that was me just a few years ago and the best advice I ever gave myself was, well, not really *advice* at all...it was a decision. I made the decision to Refuse to Diet any longer. That decision started me on the path to gaining my health back and dropping 125 pounds.

I struggled with my weight since I was a kid wearing "chubby" size clothes. I went on my first diet at age 11. This was all compounded by the fact that my mother was skinny, and had really no concept of what it was like to be chubby. She'd always been skinny, and it seemed to me that I was a poor reflection on her because I wasn't slender. Add to that, this was all happening in the 60s, at the height of Twiggy's popularity. Truth is, I look at photos of myself as a child and I appear to be a perfectly healthy, normal weight, but back then I was considered heavy, if not outright fat.

Even when I became a competitive swimmer at eleven, and later when I worked out several hours a day, I was never happy with my body. It seemed I was always trying to lose weight and yet every year I put on more. I tried all sorts of diets and I might lose a few pounds only to put it all back on, plus more.

I did this until I yo-yo dieted my way up to over 300 pounds—despite all my efforts, in fact, <u>because</u> of my efforts to lose weight, including various radical diets and hours in the gym. I don't actually know exactly how much I weighed at my peak because the scale I owned at the time stopped at 300. When I bought that scale I never dreamed I would ever come close to pegging it, but I sure did.

Not only was I fat—I was now deemed obese by my doctors. I was on medication to control heart palpitations. I was on anti-depressants.

I was told I would be on these medications the rest of my life and I needed them just so I could keep myself going day to day.

I was plagued by injuries and I was in pain pretty much all the time. I was taking pain relievers like they were candy, every day for the pain in my back, my hips and my knees. I had always been accident prone but now the injuries required surgeries. I remained as active as possible, but the strain was too much for my knees and I had surgery on both of them.

Food seemed to constantly call my name. I just looked at chocolate cake and it immediately jumped to its place on my thighs, completely by-passing the lips. Food was definitely controlling me. I hated my life and I honestly couldn't see how it was going to be better. I was only 46 years old and I was really feeling like I was destined to just get larger and larger.

So what happened? What changed in my life that allowed me to finally shed 125 pounds? What miracle occurred that gave me back my life? What magic pill, what exercise routine finally succeeded where others failed? After the pills and shakes that gave me jitters, and diets that consisted of fewer calories than a squirrel would need, what made the difference?

There was no magic pill. No exercise routine to melt away the pounds. It all started with a decision: a decision to not diet, a decision to REFUSE to diet. That single decision led to my taking control back over my life and having food go into its rightful place, as sustenance and pleasure. With this decision I have now gotten to the point where I can actually have all my favorite foods in the house and enjoy them without setting off a binge or feeling like a failure.

For the first time in my life I know that this weight loss is permanent. I have regained my health, I am off all medications, and have lost more than 120 pounds in a healthy, safe way by using my mind. That is the biggest secret that no one had ever shared with me. The power of your mind is what can make you slender. Dropping unwanted pounds of fat starts with what is in your mind. What you put into your mind has a much bigger impact on your weight than what you put into your mouth.

My personal story may be about losing over 100 pounds...but it doesn't really matter whether you have a lot to lose or if you have been struggling to lose the same 20 pounds for years...the same principles apply. The bottom line is that you can have permanent success only if you start by changing your mind first.

That is why this is not a "diet book". Changing your mind is much more than that, and it works. It works without a "diet." It works by changing your thoughts, your feelings and your beliefs. By starting there, with your inner world, it is then inevitable that your outer world will also change.

There will be people who will look at me and say that they can't learn from me because I am not a size two, or because I don't have five percent body fat and six-pack abs. I realize and accept this because I know those people are coming from their history, their experience, and their dreams and goals. Truth is, I used to want to be super slender and to have that six-pack ab type body, and if that is your goal I will not find any fault with it, as long as you aren't thwarting your health with unrealistic expectations. I know that I am a healthy weight for me and I'm able to do what I want, buy "normal sized" clothes and I feel great...that is how I measure my success— not by my weight or size, but by how I feel!

Earlier this year I was speaking with a weight loss "expert" about my book and the community that I was proposing to create. She looked at me and told me that I had to get a makeover if I was going to be taken seriously in the weight loss arena! I don't know if she is right or not, but I do know that my goal is to be my authentic self, and to help others be their authentic selves. It isn't about my appearance, it is about how I feel. OK, if I could look like Christie Brinkley I'd be thrilled, but I also know myself well enough to realize I am just not willing to put in the time that it takes! So I'm not going to have a makeover for my book photo or website and then have you meet me on the street and be shocked! One of the major reasons I gained weight in the first place is because I was trying to live up to someone else's expectations, what someone else wanted for me rather than living my true life. I'm giving that up along with refusing to diet. For me they go hand in hand, all the way to the landfill!

When we go on a diet, we set ourselves up to fail because we automatically make a diet a temporary event. "I will diet until I lose ten pounds", or twenty, or until I fit into that dress. Whatever the goal is, we may manage to stick to the diet long enough to achieve it, but then it ends. If our thoughts remain the same, then we will regain all the weight we have lost, and typically more because our habits of eating won't have changed. Our eating habits are the physical demonstration of our beliefs, our bodies are the manifestation of our beliefs, and our beliefs are merely the thoughts we have had over and over again.

Recognize that overeating can be an addiction like any other. We use food as our drug of choice to numb our feelings so we can cope or get through the day. This coping then becomes a habit. When we come out of our sugar "high" we berate ourselves for being weak, or stupid, or being a failure yet again. This just pushes us to go back to our coping mechanism, eating, setting off the vicious cycle.

Life goes on; there is no end like there is with a diet. So rather than dieting, create a new life for yourself...a new beginning where your body will settle itself into its ideal weight.

In this book, I will share with you tips and tools that I have used to successfully break the diet habit and achieve a healthy, energetic body.

What if you could lose the excess fat that you have been carrying around for years? What if you could maintain a healthy weight without struggling? I am here to tell you that you CAN. You can achieve a weight that is healthy for you, and you will find it is natural to maintain this weight. It may fluctuate a bit, but that is normal. You won't have to panic every time you put on a pound, wondering if it is all going to come cascading back.

Will it happen overnight? No. It is a process, a journey, a wonderful ride...one that I am proud to help you along. As you follow this path, pay attention to your thoughts and feelings, be willing to reset your beliefs. By changing your mind you will be changing your body. Be easy with yourself about this, there is no need to beat yourself up. You can have success this time, if you Refuse to Diet!

You'll notice there are no strings of letters after my name. I'm not a doctor, nurse, trainer, psychologist, nutritionist or dietician. I didn't go to university to study any of those things. I was actually an art major! I did go to "the school of hard knocks," aka real life experience, for my knowledge of dieting and weight loss. So what you are about to read is my experience on this journey to health.

Along the way I have met many people who do have lots of letters after their names, and I credit many of them for teaching me along my path. So I will reference people whom I have found valuable, and you can find more information about them in the Resources section at the end of the book.

There are many other wonderful teachers in the world whom I have not met, along with some "teachers" who have done more harm than good. My best advice to you is to listen to your own inner voice to help filter out those who are not helpful. Every being, even the most severely wounded, has a wise inner voice that if we would only listen will guide us to the proper teachers for us at the present moment.

I do request one thing from you: commit to finding one nugget in this book and running with it. Reading the book is not enough. If all you are going to do is read it, without even attempting to implement some of it, well then, save your money and time. The best intentions won't cut it. I have spent thousands of dollars on books, courses, exercise equipment, therapy, and trainers only to have them sit on the proverbial shelf and gather dust. This little book doesn't require anything close to that kind of commitment.

If I do say so myself there are many nuggets in this book. Commit to finding and implementing at least one. The best ideas do not have to expensive, huge, unique, difficult, or even new. Sometimes it is an old idea that we hear again, or really hear for the first time, perhaps because it is in a different context or said by a different person, or because we are now ready. Why we hear it is not important, just that we do hear it.

If you are ready and committed to finding that single nugget then I will promise that if you run with it you will see a difference in your life over time. With that success you will find other nuggets and by building up those nuggets you will create your own master jewel—you! You will be the best and brightest YOU that you can be, and I will be honored to be a part of your life.

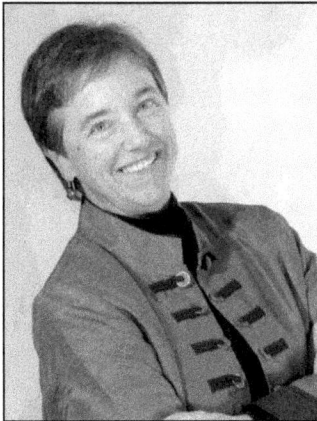

To your healthy, energetic, slender body—you deserve it!

Laurie Tossy

Chapter 2: Why Dieting is Not the Answer

"If you don't like something change it; if you can't change it, change the way you think about it."

~Mary Engelbreit

The Solution is Not a Different Diet

We try all sorts of diets, each one promising to be the answer. There are the low-carb diets, from Atkins to South Beach. Then the low-fat diets and eliminate sugar diets. My mother's favorite was the "push yourself away from the table hungry" diet. How about the anti-deprivation diet, where you stockpile your house with your favorite foods, on the theory that you overeat them because you tell yourself you aren't allowed them? There are the blood type diets and body type diets. We've measured fat grams, calories and ounces, used our hands to size up food portions at restaurants, chewed 100 times, juiced, liquefied and popped pills.

There are more diets around than you can shake a celery stick at! Some of these diets do work, for a short period of time, but you can't keep them up forever. Whether you are a student or worker or retired, an athlete or couch potato, single or married, young or middle aged or elderly, you know that diets don't work and there has got to be a better way.

Obesity Rates are on the Rise

Despite all the diets out there, despite the best intentions of the people who go on them, obesity rates in the US are on the rise. Among adults, obesity rates rose in 23 states this last year. Not a single state had a significant drop in adult obesity rates. (Source: Trust for America's Heath and the Robert Wood Johnson Foundation.)

In the past, the medical experts predicted the obese would die young and therefore not be a burden to Medicare, but these experts are now changing their tune. With every medical advance that keeps us alive longer we cost "the system" more money. Not that I am suggesting you lose weight because of financial reasons, but it is interesting to see this trend: the medical community can keep us alive longer but we remain fat and sick.

This is evidence to me that losing weight and gaining health are not the responsibility of the medical community but must rest on our shoulders. Diets seem to actually <u>increase</u> the obesity rate—people are heavier and there are more heavy people.

Why don't diets work? That is the question that people and doctors have been asking for years. The solution is not a *different* diet—the solution is to Refuse to Diet!

Weight Loss is NOT a Simple Math Equation

Have you ever been really "good" on a diet, counted every calorie, every fat gram or every carb only to find that you still weren't losing weight? I had that experience over and over, and what it proved to me is that the "simple equation" that all the doctors and scientists tell you is the answer to weight loss is not the whole story.

We are told that if we expend more calories than we take in then we have to lose weight. Unless I went through times where I expended almost no calories despite working out at the gym for over an hour every day, then I can honestly tell you the simple equation theory isn't true. There is more to it than that. I have found that sometimes our bodies will hold onto fat even though we "should" by all logic be losing weight.

How can this be? I think it just demonstrates that the mind is extremely powerful, far more powerful than most doctors know or are willing to admit. If you are not ready to lose weight permanently then your body will find a way to "hold on" to it or gain it back. That is why changing our mindset has got to be the very first step in our process for successfully and permanently losing weight.

Diets Focus on the Wrong Thing: Food

Diets don't work because they focus on food, what type of food, how much food, how often to eat, vegan, low fat, carbohydrates, liquids, etc. Naturally skinny people are not obsessed with food like the rest of us. It seems logical to me that if we want to achieve our optimum weight then we shouldn't obsess about food either.

To succeed at achieving your ideal weight you are going to have to change that focus and put it on what is going on inside your head, not what you put in your mouth! You will have to face feelings and thoughts that have been raging around and squashed down for years. If you think you can achieve a healthy body and not have to face your thoughts and feelings then you frankly are not ready, you are still looking for the magic pill or potion that will erase your fat. And that is, so not going to happen.

If just reading about facing your feelings made you reach for a pint of Ben and Jerry's or a bag of Doritos, then recognize that there is something to face. Don't beat yourself up about grabbing for your favorite treat, instead celebrate that you are being shown the real issue and the real solution—it is in your mind, not your mouth!

Dieting Teaches Us to NOT Listen to Our Bodies

We are trained to eat at a certain time, to ignore our hunger cues, to eat foods we don't enjoy.

My mother constantly told me the solution was to "push away from the table hungry"...she also made me eat dinner even if I just came home from swim practice and wasn't hungry at all. I learned to pay more attention to a clock then my own body. Granted there are times when this is useful—I couldn't expect to excel at a race for example, if I had just eaten a lot...whether I was hungry or not! And eating in class is generally not allowed, so it is normal that we govern some of our eating by the clock. But by entirely determining when to eat by the clock I totally tuned out my body's signals about hunger, pain, and discomfort. I didn't know what I wanted to eat, so I either ate what was put in front of me, or whatever was easy to grab. And typically what is easy to grab is not the healthiest food choices!

Diets are Short Term

Stories of people who have lost 30, 40, 50 or even 100 pounds are pretty inspiring, especially when they lose that weight in a really short period of time. That is what makes "The Biggest Loser" such a popular television show. It is "sexier" to be able to say "I lost 50 pounds in two months" then to say it took a year or two.

Maybe because I've done it both ways, and because I have seen so many people, myself included, have quick dramatic weight losses only to be followed by quick dramatic weight gains, these stories now just throw up red flags for me.

For one thing, I think it sets the rest of us up for comparison and failure. Sure we get the initial inspiration, but are we really following the program that the other person did? Are you working out six or eight hours a day like they do on "The Biggest Loser?" What if you do work that hard, or as hard as you can and still have a life, and you don't achieve massive results as fast as they do? Are you going to feel doubt, shame, embarrassment, hopelessness?

Fast results are often more deception that anything else, because we haven't had time to change our thinking about food and our bodies. Without those crucial changes we will not be able to maintain the weight loss. On the other hand when we change our thinking and we take consistent steps we WILL get results. Truth be told, for most of us the results will actually be faster in the long run because we won't be gaining it all back and trying to lose it over and over again...we will have a steady shift in our bodies with sustained results.

For long-term, permanent results, diets just don't work because of their very nature. They are short-term vehicles that aren't suited for the long-term journey.

Diets Don't Deal with Emotions

Our emotions and our subconscious thoughts are at the heart of the matter for most of us who are overweight, and diets don't deal with that. Diets work on the symptom, the outer manifestation, not the cause. In future chapters we will talk more about some of these thoughts, emotions and the challenges they bring, along with some tools to help us learn to deal with the challenges when they do arise!

Diets are Restrictive

By definition and tradition, diets are restrictive. Whether it is "giving up" certain foods, or limiting yourself to certain types of foods or calories, dieting feels like punishment. Even when we really want to drop some pounds, who wants to feel punished and all the thoughts and feelings that go with that?

Do you remember when you were growing up how strong the appeal was for anything that was off-limits? It might have been going somewhere or doing something, but the mere fact that we were told that it was forbidden made us want it all the more, right?

The same thing is true with food: the little kid inside will rebel if you banish all her favorite foods forever.

Food is a necessary part of living and we deserve to take pleasure in it. We may not want to indulge in overeating, any more than we would want to sleep all day and night, but we do have to eat to live.

We sleep approximately one-third of our lives but we don't set out to purposefully buy a bed that is uncomfortable so we sleep fewer hours. Instead, we acquire a comfortable bed that allows us to sleep well and wake refreshed. By getting a good night's sleep we function better when we are awake, and it is quite possible that we will need fewer hours of rest because of the quality of sleep we get.

The same philosophy can be applied to eating! Getting good quality nutrition into our bodies along with tastes that we enjoy, can give us more energy, better health and also result in our desire and need for less food!

My philosophy is there are no forbidden foods! By taking off that label I now have given myself permission to eat anything I want. That act alone takes away some of the rebellion factor and reduces number of times my "inner child" acts up and wants a treat!

Diets Deal with Illusion of Perfection

We deserve to give up the illusion that we have to be perfect, that we have to have the perfect body, that we have to be a size two (or whatever the magic size is for you,) and that we have to look like the photos in the magazines. We have to realize that those photos are illusions. Every one of those magazine shots, especially the covers, has dozens of people who are taking care of makeup, hair, clothing, lighting, posing the model, softening and sharpening of the image, adding the right amount of "wind." Then after the photo shoot, there are people who manipulate the photo with airbrushing to make the person look slimmer and remove "imperfections" like moles and freckles and shadows under the eyes.

There is no way that real people can match the illusion that is done by the magicians who work on the photo shoot and who touch it up later. The photos that are in magazines are there to sell the magazine, and as such, they are more of a piece of art than a photo of a real person. Rather than trying to achieve a false illusion of what the media tells us is "perfection" we really are better off going for being the best that we can be.

That's the beauty of humanity to me, our incredible variety. I'm 5'6" and I will never be 5'10"...that is just the way it is. I will also never, ever be a size 2—my skeletal structure just doesn't allow for that size.

Look at some of your favorite people, some of the great teachers you admire in the world. Do they match the media image of perfection? Some of them might when you see their photos on book jackets or in magazines because they, too, have gone through the magic of the photo shoot. But look at how real they are--they don't have "perfect" bodies. They are fit, they take care of themselves, but most of them don't worry about whether or not they might have an extra ten pounds on their bodies. There is a more important message they have to give, and so do you. Be the best person you can be on the inside, and when you do that, you will be the best person you can be on the outside.

It may be that you are naturally a runner, and you are going to hit your stride and will become very slender because that activity suits you, feeds you and feeds your soul. But if you are a natural writer then you might not have a runner's muscles, you will have different muscles, both literally and figuratively. You still want to take care of the body that houses that writer, because you want the energy and stamina that exercise and eating right provides, but your nature will direct you in a different avenue. For me, I have tried running and I just don't enjoy it. It doesn't feel good, and I will never have that slender marathoner's body, but I have a strong, healthy body that is good for me.

Chapter 3: Dieting, the Big Fat Lie

"Truth only reveals itself when one gives up all preconceived ideas."

~Shoseki

Lies You've Been Told about Weight

There are hundreds of different lies we have been told about weight, our bodies, and dieting. Here is a list of just some of them. Some of these are lies I told myself, others are things I've heard other people say, but I chose not to believe them personally. We all have lies that we accept as truth, and it is important that we recognize the stories we have been told so we can change the patterns. Awareness is the first step in making a change.

Family/ Genetic

I was fat as a kid, so I am always going to be fat

My parents were fat so I'm destined to be fat—it's in my genes

Success/Failure

I just can't lose weight, no matter what I try

I will never be able to eat my favorite foods again

Age/ Gender

I'm middle-aged so it is impossible for me to lose weight

It is inevitable that we gain weight as we get older

It is impossible to lose the pregnancy/baby weight

Women have to work harder than men to lose weight

Exercise

It takes a LOT of exercise to lose weight

I hate to exercise so I'll never be my ideal weight

Time

I don't have time to eat healthy foods

I don't have time to eat breakfast

I'll have to make different meals for my family and that takes too much time and planning

Moods

I will be cranky if I try to lose weight

I am nicer when I eat sugar

When I eat I feel better emotionally

Calories/ Food/Cravings

Foods call my name—I can't have ice cream (or bread or chocolate or whatever) in the house

Food cravings are a natural, healthy thing

Sugar & caffeine give me my energy I can't give them up

If I have breakfast I want more food later in the day

If I skip breakfast I am saving calories

I'll feel hungry if I try to lose weight

I'm not that hungry so I will wait and save calories

I can't eat ___ because it has too many calories

To be a healthy weight I can never have my favorite foods again

I can overeat today and starve tomorrow and it will all balance out

If I count calories and take in fewer calories than I expend I am guaranteed to lose weight

If I eat too much I can just exercise more to make up the difference

Other Health

Smoking helps you lose weight

Quitting smoking makes you gain weight, and I don't want to gain any more weight

Obesity is only hurting me, so what does it matter

> Overeating that leads to obesity does hurt others, at least in a financial sense. Obesity among baby boomers is rising and as we enter the ranks of Medicare, the cost to take care of the obese baby boomers rests with your fellow tax payers.

According to the Robert Wood Johnson Foundation it costs Medicare $1,400-$6,000 additionally per year to provide health care for an obese senior than one who is not obese. These costs include additional surgeries for things like knee replacements as well as treatments for illness such as diabetes.

In 1991 not a single state had an obesity rate over 20%. In 2009 Colorado was the only state with a rate less than 20%! Nation-wide one in three American adults is obese. (Source: The Centers for Disease Control and Prevention)

Eating is my only vice and it doesn't hurt anyone else

Eating per se, may not hurt anyone else, but if you are eating to hide your emotions you are hiding a part of yourself. By not being fully present in the world you are depriving the world of your unique self.

I can be fat without it affecting my health

People who are obese have a much greater likelihood of developing serious life-threatening diseases such as diabetes and kidney problems. In addition the excess weight leads to back problems and deterioration of hips and knees.

None of these health issues should be minimized. Severe pain obviously leads to a lower quality of life. Diabetes can lead to blindness, pain, loss of limbs and death. It isn't my goal to scare people into taking care of themselves—I don't believe that works, but it is important that we know there are consequences for our choices.

What Lies Do You Believe?

Write down the lies you have been told, you can start with my list and build from there or start from scratch. These lies are the thoughts that your subconscious has accepted as truth. You will want to change that programming in order to achieve a healthy weight permanently.

Use the worksheet in the Resources section of this book, or download a worksheet by going to my website to help you identify the lies you have accepted as truths, and how to rework them to your advantage.

http://www.RefuseToDiet.com/lies

Chapter 4: My Story, from Fat to Not

"I know God won't give me anything
I can't handle. I just wish that He
didn't trust me so much."

~Mother Theresa

Emotional Eating Starts Early

I moved a lot as a child. By the time I started kindergarten I was living in my fourth home, in my third state. I had already lived in the Midwest and both coasts by my fifth birthday. My dad worked for IBM, which we always joked stood for "I've Been Moved." Shortly after I turned eight I added living overseas to my list of addresses when my father was transferred to Japan.

This moving around led to some great skills and some less than healthy coping mechanisms. I was lonely a lot but really wasn't allowed to show it, so I ate. I learned very early that eating felt good, at least temporarily. Even my family reinforced it by giving me ice cream when I was really sad. Looking back, it was not surprising that I wasn't skinny; it was probably more surprising that I wasn't fatter than I was.

Food became my friend. I knew that food would be there even when I moved away or my friends did. Fat became a protection device. It kept people at arm's length distance. I made casual friendships pretty easily but deep friendships didn't survive long distances so friends were always viewed as temporary. Kids who moved a lot tended to gravitate towards one another, because we knew what it was like. But we also knew that one or the other of us could be moved pretty much at a moment's notice.

I developed physically pretty early. I was one of the tallest kids in my class and I was wearing a bra in the fifth grade. And, being a tall (relatively speaking) blonde in a country of short dark haired people led me to stand out in ways that I did not appreciate. I was constantly being stopped by well-intentioned Japanese people who wanted to have their picture taken with me, or wanted to practice their English "on" me. That was bad enough, but then there were the people who wanted to touch my hair—they would literally pet me on the head. This happened numerous times, each time I walked out the door.

The pressure to be "good" and to represent our country weighed heavily on my shoulders. I took the message that I was a "little ambassador" to heart and felt my every move and comment was something for which our entire nation might be judged. At the same time I absorbed the message that adults knew everything and that I was not to question what adults said or did. This turned out to be a painful combination.

Traveling in Japan was both liberating and confining at the same time. It was considered quite safe, so even as fifth and sixth graders we rode the trains and subways on our own. This was an incredibly wonderful experience and very empowering. However, the trains and subways were frequently jam packed. There were railway employees whose job it was to help push more people into the cars, wearing gloves so as to not actually touch anyone, and to also pull people out who would become so trapped in the crowded car they couldn't extricate themselves. There were numerous times when some "elastic-man" would find my arm and pull me out.

This was not a pleasant experience, but by far the worst part of it was the fact that the Japanese men seemed to have free reign to fondle my body the entire time I was in the train. My arms would be pinned to my sides; I literally could not move. I cannot tell you how many times or by how many different men my body was groped and prodded. I just know that it felt awful, dirty and shameful.

I never told anyone what was happening. I recall thinking that maybe this experience was normal, or normal for Japan, and that I was wrong for feeling uncomfortable about it.

Whether I realized it wasn't right, or feared that it was my fault, I also remember being afraid that if I told anyone what was happening, I wouldn't be allowed to go on the train alone again. The fear of losing that freedom must have outweighed my discomfort because I kept my mouth shut. The result was I didn't know what were appropriate boundaries regarding my own body. Men touched me and later men exposed themselves to me and I honestly didn't know what to do, so I ate. Later when it came time to date, I still didn't know what to do. So I ate some more.

Food and fat became my protection. But it really was a double edged sword. I felt bad so I ate. But then I felt bad because I ate, so I ate more. At a very early age I had set in motion a pattern that would take decades for me to heal.

Yo-Yo Dieting: The Ups and Downs of Weight in my Teens and Twenties

Most dieters are familiar with the yo-yo diet concept and have had the experience of losing weight only to gain it back and then repeating the process over and over. My life story is no different.

I went on my first diet at age eleven and it was a perpetual roller-coaster ride from that moment on. I went on just about every diet you could imagine. This was while I was a competitive swimmer, too. I recall being on the low carb diet in the early 1970s. I counted carb grams like Hail Marys. I allowed myself 70 grams of carbohydrate a day while I was swimming one and half hours and riding my bicycle the mile to and from the pool and then another couple miles to a different pool where I was diving for an hour.

When swimming ended for the season, I cut my carbs back to only 60 grams a day. It didn't really matter, I had hit a plateau. My best friend would have a lunch of Coca-cola and Snickers bars while I would munch carrots, dry salad and tuna fish. She was a stick and I was...well...not.

I remember the grapefruit diet and the negative calorie diet, where you were supposed to eat a bunch of foods that theoretically required more calories for your body to burn than they actually contained. I ate gallons of cabbage soup. I had apple cider vinegar in the morning.

It seemed like I would lose a little weight, but never quite enough. I remember overhearing my mother talking to her best friend, commenting how sad it was that I could never seem to lose that final ten pounds.

In junior high I had to take home economics, which scarred me for life! My teacher was bugging me about my weight. I was dieting. At the same time we were required to sew a skirt. I took the skirt in three times over the course of the semester, but because my dieting was working, at least temporarily, the skirt was too big, so I was given a C.

Whenever we took a break from swimming I would gain ten pounds back. We generally had two major breaks, one at the end of summer before school swimming started and one at winter break. Then I stopped being able to lose the ten pounds and soon I was twenty pounds overweight, then thirty and then forty.

I got to a point where I was really good at dropping and regaining twenty pounds; I could pretty much gain twenty pounds in a week. According to physics I doubt that is possible, but I saw it happen! Unfortunately it took a lot more work to lose that weight, which just never seemed fair. I had lost over 100 pounds before I graduated high school--*it was just the same twenty pounds over and over.* All dieters seem to have a certain number that their yo-yo is set at. For me it was twenty pounds. I've known people who were so tightly wound their yo-yo was set at a five pound fluctuation.

I've often wondered what compels some people to diet feverishly over five pounds and others of us have a tolerance for twenty pound swings. I don't have an answer for that, but I know that it doesn't really matter. The issues are the same, merely the numbers change.

You may have heard about Michael Hebranko. He's been on the Oprah Show a couple of times (see resources for a link for additional information.) In the late 1980s, Michael lost almost 1000 pounds. Yes, that is with three zeroes. Sadly, Michael set himself up to be the king of yo-yo dieters as he did not learn to deal with the emotional issues behind his eating. Within a few years he was back up to being more than 1000 pounds overweight. One of the things that struck me about this brave soul's journey back to health, which he is now on, is that he admits his battle is in his head. He considered having surgery but realized, "I don't get hungry in my stomach or full in my stomach. My disease is in my head, so until they invent a brain by-pass, surgery is not an option for me."

By the time I finished my freshman year in college I was fifty pounds overweight and severely depressed. That was in 1977 and I went on the radical liquid protein diet. I ended up getting down to 115 pounds at one point because of that diet, a full 25 pounds less than I had ever weighed...and significantly less than I should have weighed.

For the first time in my life I was actually skinny! This is when I learned another powerful series of lessons.

The first lesson I learned was that our *body image and actual size are not related.* I lost the weight so quickly that my brain did not have time to catch up. Not only did people at school not recognize me, I didn't recognize myself. My mother was thrilled and bought me new clothes, and for the first time it was actually fun to go shopping. I recall shopping in a little boutique in an outdoor mall in San Jose, California. I grabbed a dressy outfit just for fun, I had no place to wear it, no reason to buy it, but I wanted to see what it looked like on me because it was just so beautiful. When I came out of the dressing room I walked towards the mirrors. On the way there, another woman started walking towards me. You know the funny, awkward dance that happens as two people move to the side to pass one another, but you both move in the same direction at the same time? We did this block step several times before it sunk in that I was already at the mirror and that "other woman" was me!

My mother thought this was hilarious. I had made such a dramatic change in my body that I literally did not recognize myself in the mirror. Looking at it with my perfect 20-20 hindsight I should have known that warning bells should have been going off in my head.

This was also my first lesson about anorexia. My period stopped and my hair started to fall out. Somehow with all that, and even though my bones were sticking out and it was painful to sit, I still thought I was fat. Anorexia wasn't really known back then, but I remember the school nurse telling me I needed to gain some weight. I told her that I had to lose a couple pounds because I was going to go home for Christmas and I would gain a bunch then. That was the first Christmas in my life that I actually lost weight.

Lesson two was that guys liked skinny girls. Guys started to pay attention to me in ways they hadn't since I was a kid in Japan. Since I never learned about boundaries and how to tell somebody what was off limits this was an extremely uncomfortable period in my life. It seemed to me that all guys had at least eight arms.

On top of that, other people were treating me differently, too. People treated me like I was weak. Even my skinny best friend started protecting me.

The combination was too much for me. I started to drink, which didn't help. Fortunately for me, I didn't like the feeling of being out of control. Also fortunately for me, the guys who were around when I was drinking were protective and didn't take advantage of me. I am really grateful for that. Of course a few tried and I remember on at least one occasion bursting into tears and that stopped it. This could have been a much different story—not everyone is as fortunate.

I did get my first "boyfriend" during this time. I was19, he was 31. We dated for a while and then he started seeing someone else, someone closer to his own age and someone with some "meat on her bones."

So I started eating again. My skinny period lasted only a few months. I was in a play and I remember accusing the costumer of shrinking my costume. Of course my costume was not changing size, but I was. Again, I had no concept of what I really looked like, so I couldn't see what was happening when I looked in the mirror.

When I finally gave up yo-yo dieting I was at 300 pounds. It wasn't because I gave up dieting that I got to that weight. Certainly that is what most of us fear, but it was actually because of all the dieting that I weighed that much. Like Michael, I rarely felt real physical hunger, and if I did I pushed myself past it. I ate or didn't eat because of other external cues. Some of these were emotional reactions to forces outside myself and others where simple schedules that I "had to keep." For example, it is noon therefore I "must" eat lunch whether I am hungry of not.

Learning to Accept Myself

Of course I gained back every pound I had lost, and then added on a few more for good measure. The good thing was I didn't allow my ever increasing size to keep me from doing things. Except that I wouldn't be in photos. But that was nothing new, I rarely was photographed from the time I turned eleven.

So while I was learning to accept that I was fat, I still really had no clue what I actually looked like. Even when I was in a full length mirror my eyes couldn't be trusted. If I could see fat when I was 115 pounds, I was equally capable of seeing someone smaller than reality when I reached 190 pounds (and later 300 pounds). I avoided full length mirrors and being photographed like the plague, and when I found myself in a situation where they were unavoidable I still managed to focus on only my face or eyes.

I managed to continue this lie and the yo-yo dieting well into my thirties. I still tried dieting. I dropped another significant bunch of weight with Weight Watchers. Once again, guys seemed to like me better when I was thinner. I quickly got another boyfriend so I didn't have to worry about that pressure, and yet, I once again regained it all and then some.

I heard at some point that I needed to learn to love my body and find beauty in it and to look in the mirror and say positive affirmations about my body. This was a huge challenge for me. I could barely look at myself in the mirror to wash my face and brush my teeth. I certainly didn't think there was anything to admire about my body.

I have found this to be a very common problem for women, and it can stop them from making progress in their health, just like it did me for a long time. Our notions of beauty are so influenced by media and society that when our bodies aren't in alignment with that image we can feel ugly—no matter how much or how little we weigh.

What helped me was to shift the focus from trying to find something "beautiful" about my body, to finding things I could be grateful for about my body. I started with appreciation and gratitude which are not hindered by concepts of beauty. They are truly the precursors to love.

What attribute about your body can you appreciate? For me, I was physically strong, even though I was obese and so I was still quite active. So I started there, feeling gratitude for my strong legs that carried me around, my strong arms that pulled me through the water when I swam.

If you follow this tip, you will find as I did, that as your appreciation grows for your body you can actually start to feel the love for it. I will always have a large frame and large muscles. I am not the Miss America body type and for most of my life I focused on that and believed that meant I was ugly. I was looking at what I did not have. By turning that around and appreciating what I do have, I was finally able to get my head to be in the place where I could lose the fat. Before then I was too vested in disliking my body. I couldn't achieve a healthy weight because gee, if I did, I might actually look good and then where would I be?!

I learned you have to have feeling behind your affirmations. By feeling healthy, strong, slender, not just saying the words, then you will achieve the result. It was a big stretch for me to think I could feel slender at 300 pounds, but with every pound lost I could feel the comparative slenderness, and more importantly, I could feel my improving health and energy.

"Say you are well, or all is well with you,

And God shall hear your words and make them true."

~Ella Wheeler Wilcox

Chapter 5: Finding the Answer

> "By accepting responsibility for my results, I claim my power."
>
> ~Laurie Tossy

It Starts with Changing Your Mind.

Where does everyone place the emphasis when looking at dropping weight? Whether it is five pounds or fifty, we have been taught to focus on the external results, what we look like, and the specific plan, the "diet" or the exercise routine. This is like a two-legged stool. You might be able to balance on it for a while, but at some point you are just going to fall over!

Instead of that balancing act, it is critical we build a really strong foundation and rise from that. Envision a pyramid. The bottom third, the base, is your foundation, which is all about your decision, your mindset, your commitment to being the healthy person you can BE.

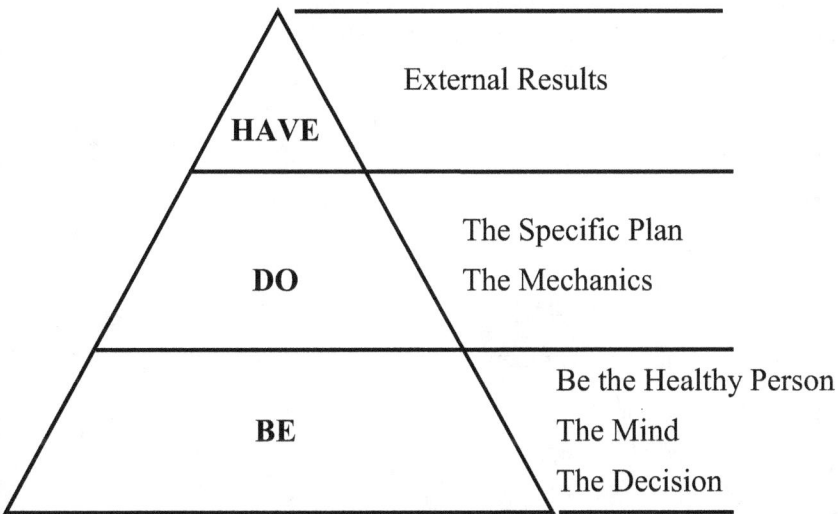

```
        /\         _____
       /  \        External Results
      / HAVE\
     /_____\
    /        \     The Specific Plan
   /   DO     \    The Mechanics
  /_____\
 /              \  Be the Healthy Person
/      BE        \ The Mind
/_____\ The Decision
```

Moving up the pyramid is the specific plan or elements to your process. These are the things you are going to DO. It may be changing foods you eat, chewing each mouthful 12 times (remember that one? I think it was invented by the same person who told us to brush our hair 100 strokes each night!) This is the mechanics, so it includes any exercises you are going to do, whether you tell other people about your plan or keep it a secret.

The apex of the pyramid can only be attained after the base and middle sections are set. This is the end result and it will occur pretty much on its own because you have already built the majority of the pyramid. This is what you HAVE at the end.

Your pyramid is Be, Do, Have. You can't Have the end results by Doing first, you have to BE first and then you can Do and then Have. Rather than focusing on your two-legged stool, focus on your decision and you will naturally build your full pyramid and have the results you desire.

Who Do You Want to Be?

When I was struggling with my weight I didn't like myself very much. I tried to be a good person but I felt so out of control I didn't like ME and I thought that if anyone knew "the truth about me" they wouldn't like me either.

In the midst of all this I somehow decided that I had had enough. I decided I was not going to take it anymore and I was going to reach out and grab my life. I decided I would be the best ME I could, even if that person didn't seem like much to anyone else. So I thought about what I wanted in life, the type of person I wanted to be and I made a list.

- I wanted health

- I wanted happiness

- I wanted life...to live

- I refused to roll over and die

- I realized I had not failed at dieting but diets had failed me

- I decided I would succeed

- I would achieve

- I deserved success

- I refused to punish myself with restrictions, limitations, guilt trips and injuries

- I refused to diet

Decide what you want in your life, the type of person you want to be. Make your list and use it as the foundation for your pyramid. Again, a worksheet is available in the Resources section of this book, or you can go to my website and download a worksheet that will help you in building your own list, http://www.RefuseToDiet.com/desires

My Mind Was My Biggest Obstacle

> "The greatest discovery of my generation is that a human being can alter his life by altering his attitudes."
>
> ~William James

I realized that my mind was the biggest obstacle to my success and that it could also be my greatest asset. When I say "mind" I am not talking about "willpower," it is about changing my thinking. It is actually more important to focus our attention and energy on what is going on inside our minds than what we are placing in our mouths. When we focus on our minds we automatically begin to adjust our eating and exercise habits.

We start by changing our inner world, by looking within for love and approval rather than seeking if from outside.

When I realized my being fat had more to do with what was going on in my head than what was going in my mouth it was an "ah ha" moment. It wasn't a light bulb moment, it was an entire paparazzi of flashes that illuminated my soul for the briefest time.

In order to get rid of my excess fat I had to realize and accept that I was the one who made me fat. No one else. Not my mother, not my genes, not society, not the media, not illness, not injury, not the guys in Japan. I was completely responsible. What was surprising to me was how liberating it was to realize that, because when I realized I was responsible, it meant I also had the ability to change it.

Sure there were some outside influences, but every choice I made that was unhealthy was my choice. Including the times when I chose to listen to the outside influences. This realization was the beginning of a wonderful new fork in my journey. I'm not going to claim perfection, in fact that is no longer my goal. What I do claim is I am making better health choices and my body is reflecting those choices. By accepting responsibility for my results I claim my power.

There's no Dr. Frankenstein ready to do a brain transplant that will solve this situation for you. Nope, it is going to take some work on your part. This is where you can take the list of lies that you have accepted, rework those into positive thoughts—some real truths, and start to change your life! If you haven't already done so, create your list of lies and start working on them one by one. Refer to Chapter 3 if you need to refresh your memory.

Mind vs Emotions

Our minds got us here and our minds will get us out. A key point to consider is there is a large distinction between our minds and our emotions. Emotions just are. They happen and as much as we want to, we cannot control our emotions. This was a huge light bulb moment for me. I started to have a real weight problem just about the time I hit puberty, about the same time that I started trying to control my emotions. The way I tried to "control" them was to turn them off or shut them down, which really meant to tune them out any way I could...to ignore them.

We can't control our emotions but we can control how we react and whether or not we let them control us. Esther Hicks in the teachings of Abraham and the book *Ask and It is Given,* tells us we can reach for better feeling thoughts, but that we cannot just ignore our emotions. We can only have one emotion or feeling at a time and we can continually work at keeping better feeling thoughts present. This is a great book with different exercises for learning to feel better, to raise our emotional vibration. Check your local library, bookstore or you can order by going to http://www.RefuseToDiet.com/askabraham.

Facing your emotions does not mean you will become a raving lunatic or a shrew or that people will wonder if it is "that time of the month." Our fear of how people will react to our expressing our emotions is one of the key reasons we numb our feelings in the first place. Have you ever feared you would over react and just explode? I used to be afraid I would get so angry that I would literally hurt someone.

I remember one time when I was about twelve—I smacked someone on the back in greeting—I wasn't angry, just energetic—and that action left a welt on my friend's back. That experience demonstrated that I could actually hurt someone by expressing myself...by just being me. If I could hurt someone when I wasn't even mad, imagine what I could do if I was truly angry! My imagination was as powerful as that smack, and left a huge welt on my soul, and I began to pull back...and to eat.

My own anger scared me so much I refused to allow myself to admit to it, to feel it. So I numbed myself to it. Then I would become angry at myself for overeating and I had to numb that anger out too.

I had a warped concept that it was okay to be angry at myself, to hate myself, but it was not okay to be angry at anyone else. I have since learned that is a very common thought process for women. It just isn't acceptable for women and girls to express anger. I believe that is one of the reasons women often cry when we get angry. Even though this is frustrating to our loved ones who happen to be born with a Y chromosome, it has been drummed into our heads that it is okay for us to cry but not to yell.

Anger may not be your hot button, it might be joy or fear, or a combination of them. For many of us we seem to be able to only handle a certain amount of emotion of any kind. Any more than that threshold sends us running to the M&Ms.

Think of your emotions like a graph, where they are either positive or negative, not meaning good or bad, merely above or below the baseline.

Positive
(joy, love, etc.)

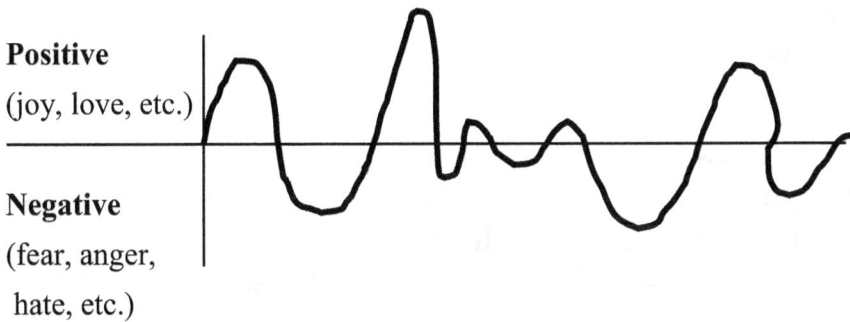

Negative
(fear, anger,
 hate, etc.)

As human beings we have a full range of emotions. Most of us are much more accepting of those we label "positive", those above the line, such as joy, love, happiness, and we are less tolerant of "negative" emotions like fear and anger. So instead of our graph showing the full range of emotions, we try to control it and we want it to look more like this:

Positive

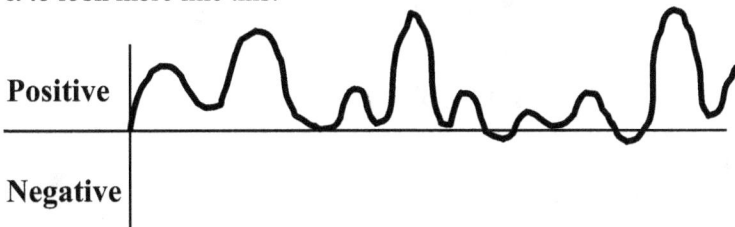

Negative

There are some people who can't handle the "positive" emotions and their emotional graph will be the opposite.

Other people realize that there is a yin and yang to life and so they know that experiencing bliss all the time is not going to happen. So they look for a flatter more calm experience like this:

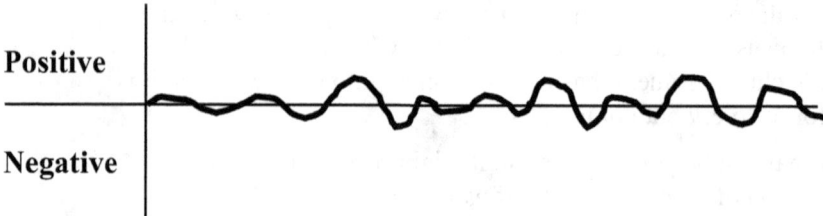

Positive

Negative

Neither of these last two graphs are realistic nor healthy for most of us. Perhaps a Buddhist Monk can achieve them, but I'm better off accepting that I have a full range of emotions...besides I look terrible in orange!

The truth is our emotions are neither positive nor negative, good nor bad, they just are. The sooner we realize and accept that, the more quickly we can progress.

"When you think you've accepted all your emotions you will be given lots of opportunities to test that theory."

~Laurie Tossy

Remember this is not a competition, this is a journey. You are going to feel things and you will want to reach for your drug of choice and sometimes you will grab hold of it and other times you will let it be. I realized I was well on my way to a full "recovery" when a friend of mine died and I didn't reach for ice cream, cookies or alcohol to cover up the feelings. I let myself be with the emotions and I really felt fully human even as my heart felt broken. This was a huge milestone for me.

If you think you've realized and accepted all your emotions, in all their glory, you'll be given lots of opportunities to test that theory. Two years ago I was tested further when my father died. I went on an eating spree that lasted for a couple months. Sometimes things seem too painful for us to endure, so we get through them the only way we can. If/when this happens to you, be gentle with yourself and remember you are doing the best you can at that moment. Don't make it worse by berating yourself for falling back on your old patterns. You also don't have to let the old patterns take complete control. At some point you will, like me, say to yourself "How long am I going to let this go on? How long will I allow this to be my excuse to not be healthy?"

If we don't have control over our emotions and yet, generally speaking, we don't want to rage, rail or cry in front of our co-workers, boss, neighbors or kids, what do we do? We do have control over our reactions to our feelings and this is key. Our minds got us into this mess because our minds are where we act or react. We can <u>react</u> to our feeling by overeating, thereby numbing that feeling or we can choose to <u>act</u> in a different way. In other words we have a choice. We have control! We have power!

Create a List of Alternate Reactions

This is a new concept for most of us and we will need to develop some new skills in order to control our reactions to our emotions. Before you go "cold turkey" you will want to set up some alternate ways to act that will help you get through various emotions. I've listed a few ideas that I've used, but your list may be different.

Take some time to create your own list. Write your thoughts down on a clean piece of paper that you can refer back to. You might want to laminate it and put it on the fridge or cupboard. Whatever you do, do not bury it. This is a tool you will want to refer to often, especially in the beginning. I like sleeve protectors rather than laminating because then I can add to it as new ideas and skills emerge. You want to have lots of things on this list. Some will be tools you can use in public and others will be things that you prefer to do in private. Some will work better for you with one emotion and or how intensely you are feeling an emotion.

Things I Can Do When I feel Emotional [rather than eating]

- Primal Scream
- Silent Primal Scream
- Go for a walk around the block
- Swim or "water walk" really hard

- Meditate
- Count to 100
- Count backwards from 100
- Curl up in a ball
- Cry
- Sleep
- Go for a drive in the country
- Listen to music and crank it up loud
- Watch a movie where it is "okay" to cry
- Ride a roller coaster
- Play with a puppy
- Seek out a baby
- Go to a park and swing
- Dance
- Laugh, at a movie, a book...
- Talk to a friend
- Write
- Paint or Sculpt
- Hit my pillow
- Hammer a nail into a board
- Vacuum
- Throw rocks into a lake
- Have a cup of coffee or tea

Did you notice that I didn't include things on my list like "go shopping"? Shopping can be just another addiction, another habit gone awry, so I will encourage you not to have shopping on your list. Window shopping is fine if that works for you, but you don't want to have your bank account get too skinny and your closets bursting at the seams during this process. We're not looking to get healthy by substituting a different habit; we are looking to achieve health through conscious choice.

A sample worksheet is available in the Resources section. Or go to my website and download the worksheet to help you create your own list:

http://www.RefuseToDiet.com/options

This is Your Plan, Use It

Now that you have your list of options, review it, highlight or star those things you believe will work the best for you. If there is anything you require in order to use that process go ahead and get it so you are ready. For example, if you were to choose "hammer a nail into a board", have a board, hammer and some nails ready! If going for a walk is a good choice for you, then have comfortable shoes wherever you'll need them. Keep a pair at work and another pair by the front door. Make it easy to engage in the new behaviors until they become the natural response.

A comment on the Primal Scream—this is an out loud, blood curdling thing that I'm just not that comfortable with and find it highly overrated. However, it works for lots of people, and it is mentioned by so many therapists that I have included it here. Maybe I am still too uptight (!) but I just imagine someone hearing me and that thought alone is enough to shove the feeling down with a Blizzard. However, the *silent* primal scream works for me because I can get my entire body into it and whether I'm in my bedroom, the closet or a washroom stall no one else knows what is going on!

I love to go for drives as a way to lift my spirits and I have several routes that I have preplanned so I know I won't start off driving by the Dairy Queen.

Sometimes a physical activity is really helpful; just pick things that you can do without hurting yourself or others. I can vacuum when angry but I don't dare attempt to dust. I can throw rocks into a lake, but I don't try to skip them because that is too frustrating. I don't try to build things that require control when I'm upset but I can have a "throw away" board and pound away at it with a few pennies in nails for cheap therapy.

You might have to try a variety of things before you find one that feels right. Sometimes quiet is the answer for me, either gentle music or nature sounds, other times I just want to rock out. I write a lot and it is a way to get some really angry, ugly stuff out, which believe me—we all have. I write it out, sometimes in huge letters, sometimes over and over again. Then I burn it or shred it so I know no one else will ever read it, including myself. I got it out of my system and I don't want to pollute myself by re-ingesting it. I find the thoughts that come out at these times are only partially true and temporary. Thoughts we all go through, like hating our partners, our parents, our God. Let yourself go through it, experience it and come out on the other side alive.

To my knowledge no one has ever been struck down for saying "I hate you" but I do recommend you say it in private or write it down and then destroy it. Saying it out loud to your mother, partner or child could have major consequences. God is more forgiving in my experience! So if you say it or scream it do it where no human can hear you.

Fatigue Can be a Side Effect

Don't be surprised if you experience some fatigue while you are making these changes. My logic told that because I was feeding my body better and shedding pounds I would have more energy. That makes sense and works to a certain degree, but you are also learning a new skill and that uses a lot of energy.

Another reason for the fatigue is you are taking in fewer stimulants. I used to keep myself awake by eating. Late night study sessions accompanied by a package of Oreos. It was very unconscious eating but it helped me get through those chapters. Or I would eat just so I could stay awake. I forced myself to stay awake until I literally crashed, so I would be so exhausted I didn't have to face my emotions even in my dreams. In the middle of the afternoon I would have soda or cookies to pump me back up. Fewer calories and stimulants can in the short term lead to less energy. Trust that this will work itself out pretty quickly and you will actually have more energy in the long-run.

Processing your emotions can lead to fatigue too, so again, be gentle with yourself as you make these changes. Just don't use that as an excuse to sleep all day every day as just another way to hide from your emotions.

You have your list, and any tools you need to activate your plan. Now you are ready. Be gentle with yourself: Rome wasn't built in a day and we didn't get fat in one either! We learned our old behaviors over time and we will learn our new healthy behaviors over time also.

Finally Choosing to Believe in the Possibility

If you accept that your mind got you into this situation and therefore only your mind can get you out of it, where do you go from here? The first step is to make the decision, "I am changing my mind. I am changing my body. I am changing my life." Then you must add, "I am worth it!" Say that over and over again every day until you can say it without feeling like a liar, because I know for most of us that is exactly how it feels in the beginning.

"What is possible? What you will."

~Augustus William Hare and Julius Charles Hare,
Guesses at Truth, by Two Brothers, 1827

Using Your Mind to Lose Weight

"You do not become good by trying to be good but by finding the goodness that is already within you and allowing that goodness to emerge. But it can only emerge if something fundamental changes in your state of consciousness."

~Eckhart Tolle, *A New Earth,*
Awakening to Your Life's Purpose

This quote really speaks to me because he emphasizes the necessity of changing our mindset, our state of consciousness in order to find what we have inside ourselves but what we have allowed to remain hidden.

In fact, I believe this thought can be applied to our bodies and our health goals, too, "You do not become slender (or strong or healthy) by trying to be slender but by finding the slenderness that is already within and allowing that slenderness to emerge, but it can only emerge if something fundamental changes in your state of consciousness"

In other words, you have to change your mindset so that you allow your natural state of good health, that is already within you, to come out and shine.

One of the keys to help you lose weight, or make any positive changes in your life, is to program your mind to think in new ways. Daily affirmations are a great tool to accomplish that.

Affirmations: What They Are, Why They Work, Why People Think They Don't

Affirmations are generally thought of as positive, but really all an affirmation is, is a series of words, a thought that you repeat, that you affirm. Any thought can be an affirmation. We make thoughts firm by repeating them over and over.

An affirmation is not inherently positive or true, in fact the reason we tend to think of affirmations as positive is because that is the type of affirmations we are taught to make <u>now</u> to correct all the messages we have given ourselves in the <u>past</u>.

An affirmation, used as a tool, is a positive statement written in the present tense, first person. This affirmation must be repeated over and over. That is why a lot of people don't believe affirmations work. They think that there is something magical in the positive phrase they just learned, and that by saying it once or twice every morning it will automatically come true. The real reason we have to practice positive affirmations is because we don't really believe them! If we already believed them, we wouldn't need to practice them...they would already be true!

Negative thoughts are a kind of affirmation, too. How many different negative thoughts do you have about yourself in a day? How often do you catch yourself repeating the same negative thought? Negative affirmations on the other hand, <u>these</u> we believe and have lots of practice with! We are really good at those and the only practice we need there is being aware that we are saying or thinking them and stopping! We all have negative thoughts and self-doubts from time to time. What is important is for us to move away from the negative and move toward the positive.

I find short statements to be best for affirmations: they are easier to remember! Affirmations can be said in the morning as you are waking up and at night before you fall asleep. This helps them sink into your subconscious because you are closer to that state at these times.

Mark Victor Hansen, co-author of the *Chicken Soup for the Soul* series of books suggests you give yourself "thought commands" before you go to sleep. Basically he is suggesting you set your intention for the next day and make positive affirmations as you lie in bed and are drifting off to sleep. By doing this you are putting positive information into your subconscious and giving it time to go to work. You will wake up with your subconscious having worked on processing that information, even if you are not consciously aware of the process or result.

You can also say your affirmations throughout the day. Keep a list of affirmations handy, or memorize a few key ones that you can repeat throughout the day. Place affirmations on your monitor, your bathroom mirror, in your office or in your car. Put them anywhere as a reminder to instill these positive thoughts into your subconscious

Here are some health related affirmations you can use, you can download affirmations by going to the website http://www.RefuseToDiet.com/affirmations, or refer to the resources section of the book for additional affirmations sources.

- I desire healthy foods.

- I love myself and take care of my body.

- I make healthy food choices easily.

- I move my body effortlessly throughout the day.

- I exercise joyfully on a regular basis.

- I am open to the possibility that I can achieve my ideal body weight.

- I have perfect health.

- My body burns fat efficiently.

- I am aware of what I eat.

- I choose foods that fuel my body

- In every moment I love myself where I am and I have the potential to be even better.

If you find yourself negating what you are saying, keep repeating the affirmation...or try one that you can say without having any negative responses. Be sure to keep your thoughts positive as you drift to sleep.

Mona Lisa Schultz, MD, Ph.D., physician, medical intuitive and author, suggests we do affirmations like repetitions at the gym.

Instead of lifting barbells, repeat ten times, "I love myself just the way I am"

Repetition Builds Strength

This is true not only when we are talking about physical strength, but also emotional, spiritual and mental strength as well.

Set out to learn the basic skill first so you have a good foundation. Any teacher or coach knows that it is easier to have a student improve upon a good skill than to have to unlearn a habit developed by improper application of a skill.

Then practice, practice, practice this skill until it is 2nd nature and you no longer have to think about it. In school for example, you might have used flash cards to memorize facts and figures. If you play an instrument, you practiced hand position, chords and scales before you played anything that sounded much like music. In sports, you practiced the basic components of the game—passing, receiving, the start, the turn, hitting the ball, whatever were key elements to your sport.

As you gain confidence and ability in one skill, you can learn another.

Then you can link those skills together.

Once you are solid in the basic skills then you can work to improve them. This may be by doing more repetitions (think of lifting weights for example.) Or it may be to push to go faster…whether it is running around a track or picking up the tempo on a piece of music. Perhaps it is to go for a longer period of time—for example, last week I walked for 15 minutes every day, this week I will walk for 20 minutes.

Another way to grow a skill is the amount of emotion or mental energy you put behind it. This can be viewed as the intensity of your desire, the scope of your dream. If you are half-hearted about what you are doing, you will probably get half-hearted results. However if you do the exact same level of work with passion and conviction you will get bigger results, much more quickly.

What does all this have to do with weight loss? A lot! There are some fundamental skills that you need to know in order to succeed. Affirmations are one of those skills. Of course some basic nutritional knowledge and ability to increase your physical activity are also skills to cultivate.

Think of the affirmations as the first basic skill that you are developing to reach your goal. In this case, you aren't learning to play golf or the piano you are learning to lose weight. Affirmations are like playing scales.

Practice your affirmations until you no longer stumble over the words. Know them so you can say them at any time of the day.

Once you have the confidence in knowing the words, you can work on linking different affirmations together, or adding affirmations to your repertoire. And you can practice them while you do other things—like walking or during meal prep.

Then be very aware of your words and the meaning behind the words. Visualize the end goal while you say your affirmations. Have the conviction in your heart that this is true and works.

What happens to many of us is when we don't see immediate results we say it doesn't work, when in reality we may not have given it enough time. The key is repetition and to integrate the change into our lives so time works for us!

The thought process behind affirmations is very important. In quantum physics all possibilities already exist. We can choose to identify the one we want and bring it into our reality. To do this we have to feel it, either by loving the idea or fearing it. If that thought has no feeling energy behind it, no emotions attached to it then it will not come about.

Affirmations are not something you do for a minute and then put away. Be clear about what you want to have, feel the feeling of it, and repeat it throughout the day.

We have ample opportunity for negative thoughts to dominate our minds if we allow them to...because we hear or read about standards for beauty and health...because we compare ourselves to others... or we relive moments from our past.

Whether your negative thoughts are about not being able to stick to your healthy eating goals, or how big your hips are, or how thin your lips are, or that you are lazy... or unlovable... unworthy... ugly... these thoughts do not serve you.

The good news is that you can change your thinking.

The second step to an affirmation is the emotion behind that affirmation. To really work, you need to do more than just repeat the affirmation over and over by rote. You must put some feeling behind it. One of the best ways to generate emotional power behind an affirmation is to take action that supports the affirmation. Affirmation plus action equals manifestation. That is the "magic" equation.

Affirmation + Action = Manifestation

When you first do an affirmation it may feel fake or silly. That is because it is not necessarily true at the moment, it is something you <u>want</u> to be true, but you are saying it in the present tense. It is a truth that you are drawing to yourself.

Negative Affirmations

> "Anything you complain about
> repeatedly is something you have an
> unconscious desire to reproduce"
> Gay Hendricks, author and
> co-founder of Spiritual Cinema Circle

Any time you find that you are saying something negative about yourself—your body, what you just ate, what you did or did not do for exercise—ask yourself if this is something you want to manifest in your life. If it is not, then counteract it with your positive affirmations.

You can use a negative association to help break your negative affirmation habit...put a rubber band around the wrist and snap it whenever you notice a negative thought. This gives a small uncomfortable sensation.

Or you can simply say "cancel that thought" or "that thought no longer serves me".

Immediately follow that negative association with a gentle loving sensation ("positive reinforcement") which could be as simple as rubbing the wrist gently or lightly tapping your chest while you say a positive affirmation.

Use your affirmations and combine them with positive reinforcements and tip the affirmation scale in your favor!

Affirmations and the Mirror

Louise Hay in *You Can Heal Your Life* talks a lot about affirmations and I use a lot of her suggestions myself. One of the things she says is that a "good general affirmation" is powerful and she suggests the following, "I love you ____ (your name), I really love you." Louise says that she really likes people to do affirmations in the mirror where you can look in your eyes. You know the saying that "the eyes are the window to the soul." Looking in your eyes is a way to connect with the deepest part of you, your inner child, and to reassure that child that she is loved. By looking in your eyes as you say affirmations you can also notice if saying the affirmation makes you uncomfortable or if it is easy to do.

I definitely found myself <u>very</u> uncomfortable with the whole process. It was a HUGE challenge for me. I didn't like looking at myself in the mirror at all, not even to wash my face, so the idea of looking right into my eyes and saying nice things about myself was distressing to say the least. I kept hearing a little voice in my head calling me a liar, telling me I didn't love myself, that I wasn't worthy of being loved, that I was fat and ugly and no one in their right mind would ever love me.

I have found that lots of people, especially people who are overweight, have very similar reactions to this process. After all, we are more accustomed to beating ourselves up than loving ourselves.

So I took Louise's concept and modified it in a couple key ways. This helped me to accept and even believe the love affirmations and it can help you, too. You can still have success if you skip this and choose to hear that little voice telling all those hateful lies, but it will take longer...and frankly, why put up with it? It is time to quiet that voice and replace it!

Here's what you do...find a photo of yourself as a child. Choose one that you can look at with only positive or neutral feelings. In other words, find a photo from an era before you began to criticize yourself, a photo where you can look at it and feel love for that child or infant.

Tape that photo at eye level on your mirror. Look at the photo and repeat the "I love you" affirmation. Repeat the affirmation and look back and forth between the photo and your current reflection, looking in your eyes as a child and your eyes today.

Practice this every day. Make the connection in your mind between that lovable child and you as the adult you currently are. That's why I want you to focus on your eyes because they help you connect to your soul, that inner energy. When you start this process, focus on the irises and pupils of your eyes, peering deep into your core. This is not the time to notice your physical "imperfections"

Your soul knows you are the same being as that innocent, loving and lovable child.

As you become comfortable saying "I love you" to yourself, place your hands on your chest as you say the affirmation so you physically feel the words vibrate as well as seeing the emotion in your eyes. This gives you a kinesthetic or tactile event which adds to the visual and auditory experience. By maximizing the senses involved, we reach different parts of our brain. People tap into the emotional centers in different ways, so by having all these senses activated we better assure that connection.

Once you get pretty comfortable saying "I love you" and feeling the vibration, on one of your repetitions change your focus so you look at your entire face. Gradually work up to five repetitions alternating between the deep eye focus and overall face focus.

Don't rush this process. It will take several days, possibly weeks or even months. There is no time table, no "right" length of time. The important thing is for you to be comfortable with the previous step before progressing.

The next step is to visually take in your body. Again start with one repetition, the first repetition have deep eye focus, then your face, third deep eye, then fourth entire body, fifth-10th in the series go back to deep eye and face, and the photo of the child can be interspersed in the mix, too.

As you increase the entire body focus affirmations, if you notice any hesitation on the next repetition go right to the deep eye focus and keep your focus there until you are comfortable again, even if it is for the rest of the set.

When you are doing these affirmations it is normal to have your progress vary...some days you may feel like you really need to stay on the deep eye focus and not look at your body at all—even if you had "progressed" to being able to look at your body before. Our feelings are not on a fixed straight path, so just because one day you can be confident with the process doesn't mean that you will never have times of discomfort with it. Remember that little child and connect with her.

As overweight people, we are typically not used to looking at our bodies with love—if we look at them at all. So it is important that you connect with your soul by way of the deep eye focus between the body scans.

When I talk about being "comfortable" looking at your body while repeating the love affirmations, that doesn't mean you have to believe it 100%. You may still have some level of doubt, but as long as you are not recoiling or unwilling to look at your body, you are planting the seeds.

Once you are comfortable looking at your body and stating the good, general love affirmations you can add some new affirmations. I suggest these, but you can use other affirmations that you find in the Resource area or from Louise Hay or other sources.

- I am willing to change
- I am willing and able to change
- My body aligns with its perfect and natural health

Success Tool: Take Your Photo

"The pictures you hold of yourself in your mind today have only to do with your past. If you don't take charge and create new pictures of yourself, you will only repeat tomorrow what you have done today and yesterday."

~Claude Bristol, *TNT The Power Within You*

Bristol wrote this in 1954 but it was true long before then and will remain true forever. What pictures are you holding on to? Are they accurate? Do you want to keep that picture in your brain's "photo album?" Or would you rather create a new set of images that you can enjoy for the rest of your life, starting today? You have the power. In fact, you are the only one who does have the power to change those pictures in your mind.

I didn't like having my photo taken. I hadn't since I was about 11 or 12, about the time I went on my first diet. I actually convinced myself that I would break the camera because I was so ugly. By not being photographed I gave myself the opportunity to not see myself in any objective light. So my brain held this self-image of Laurie as a strong, albeit big girl, a competitive swimmer who was a bit overweight, even though I was in my forties and weighed more than 300 pounds.

Photos are inanimate and so they give you the chance to leisurely look at your body in a way that you cannot in a mirror. And because they are fixed, the eyes are not engaged as much and so it is harder to stay focused on them. How many times have you seen a photo of yourself and been shocked at how you looked? It is like hearing a recording of your voice, we never sound like ourselves because we normally hear our voice as it resonates within our own head. It is the same thing with our body. We have a perception of what we look like and a photograph challenges that perception. Good! Challenging that perception is one of the first steps to changing it!

Develop a new set of "prints" in your mind's eye of what you look like. Get rid of the old images that are based on the past and live into your new pictures.

Take Your Photo Part 2

"No matter what your body's appearance
is on the outer level, beyond the outer
form it is an intensely alive energy field."

~Eckhart Tolle, *A New Earth,
Awakening to Your Life's Purpose*

We are going to take a look at our body and see what it looks like on the outer level and then see if we can get beyond that to feel that alive energy field inside.

Grab your camera, preferably a digital one. You are going to want to print out a large copy and you don't want anyone else to see this. This is strictly a tool for you to help you visualize yourself the way you want to look and feel. If your camera has a timer on it you can do this by yourself, otherwise enlist the help of a really good friend, a really, really good friend, someone you will allow to see your body, sagging belly and cellulite and all.

Hmmm...I think the sales of digital cameras with timers just went up!

You can wear your bra and underwear for this or a swimming suit, but avoid tanks as they can hide some of the fat and for this to work best it has got to "all hang out" quite literally. Get as much of you in the picture as possible, preferably from head to toe, but you be sure to include your head and at least to the top of your knees.

Take three pictures: front, back and side views. Stand in front of a neutral background so you stand out and aren't camouflaged in anyway. Print out these photos on regular 8.5 x11 paper, one photo per page. This is documentation, not art. Be sure the pictures are completely dry before you proceed.

Look at these pictures and realize that it is truly you. Yes, you really look like that and no, the camera didn't add ten pounds, every pound is there because of choices you made. Do you feel like that picture looks? I didn't! Most people feel either bigger or smaller than they really are, so this can be an eye opening experience.

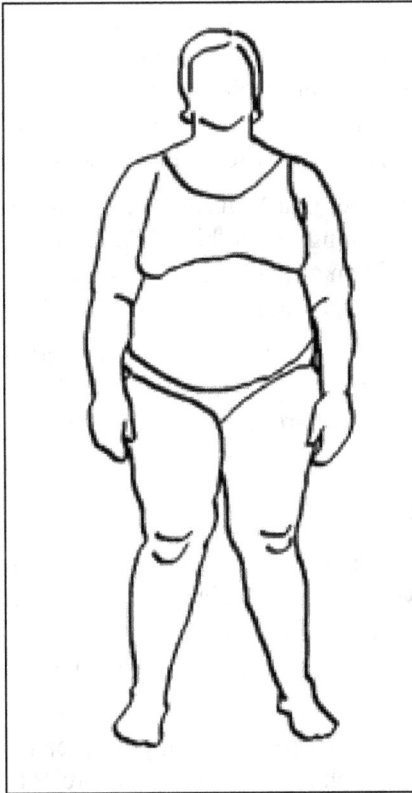

I suggest you keep a copy of the photos in your computer with the date. That way you will have a record of your starting point and you can see the transformation that happens as you shed fat.

Take as long as you need to become aware of your body and to accept it as it is. Your body is incredible! It carries you around, it breathes, digests food, allows you to read, write and do all sorts of things. Appreciate your body and accept it. Once you do that you can work on changing it. Permanent change comes from acceptance not hate. As long as you hate or feel disgust for your body you are going to be challenged to change it. Accepting your body as it is does not mean that you do not want to improve it!

If you are stuck in negativity get out another clean sheet of paper and write down all your positive attributes. Are you any less kind because you are fat? Of course not! Are you funny, generous, a good mother, a hard worker, loyal? Are any of these things dependent upon your being fit or fat? Of course not! Now take all those attributes, all those good qualities and apply them to an imaginary person "X". Look at the photo of yourself and imagine that it is a photo of "X". On another piece of paper write down what shedding fat will do for "X". If "X" is kind to animals she could enjoy them more by being able to be more mobile. If she is a good mother she would enjoy being able to pick up her children or take them to the beach. If she is generous and gives time and money to various charities then she will have more energy to do this good work.

You get the idea. Now, remember that YOU are "X". You deserve to improve your health and live a long life, to be able to keep up with your kids, to fit comfortably in an airplane seat to visit your grandkids, to be able to walk all day in a national Park or Paris.

Once you have accepted your body and feel comfortable saying "I deserve optimum health! I deserve to pay attention to me!" Now it is time to get a Sharpie and move to Part 3!

Tools: Your Photo Part 3

I learned this trick from Michael Thurmond and it works really well. You are going to draw on your picture so that you can see that person beneath the fat, to help reveal that inner energy field. This will help you in visualizing the you who is emerging from your cocoon.

Draw a line over the areas you want to cut out of your life. The great thing about using your photograph is that you see you are not going to magically transform into Angelina Jolie, it helps you to see your basic body structure. Draw the outline of your new silhouette keeping your body structure in place. Now add some cross hatches to minimize what is outside the line but don't "paint" it all out. Now you have a set of pictures where you can see your core self more prominently and you can also still see yourself as you are physically today.

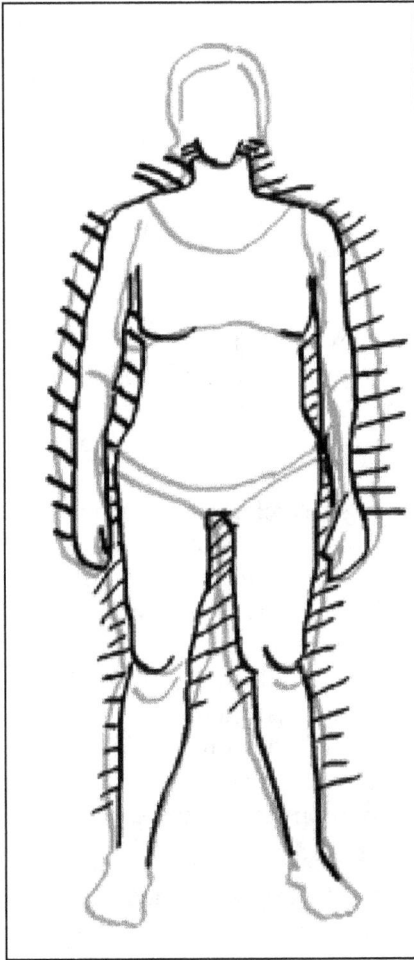

Take these pictures and put them in sleeve protectors and have them where you can refer to them often.

Getting Clear on the Goal and "the Why"

It is important to get clear on what your goals are and why. What is your goal when it comes to your health? What prompted you to read this book?

- Do you want to drop excess fat? It might be 10 lbs, 20 lbs, 50 lbs, 100 lbs or more

- Do want to improve your health? Maybe have less fat and better fitness?

There are no wrong answers, just know what you general goal is.

Why do you want to lose weight?

You may think it is strange to ask yourself this question, but I assure you it is critical to your health goal success: why do you want to lose weight? Seriously, this is not a rhetorical question. There are lots of reasons for wanting to drop pounds and there really aren't any "wrong" reasons, but there are a lot of incomplete ones.

When you think about why you want to drop weight, pay close attention to your language. Are you focusing on "losing" weight? Bob Proctor claims that as long as we use words like "lose" weight we are really looking to find it again. Losing something implies that it is a sad situation that we want to end or to find that item again. After all, we lose our keys and go searching to find them. We are sad when we lose a parent. To lose has all sorts of negative connotations, elections are lost; people lose faith in one another. So consider the possibility of using different terminology. That is a huge challenge, one that I'm not always successful at, because "losing weight" is deeply ingrained in our vocabulary. If this is an "ah ha!" for you then think about a term that feels better, seems more permanent, or easy to accomplish than "losing weight". Sometimes a simple shift in language can make a huge difference. Perhaps you want to take off excess weight, shed some fat or drop those pounds.

Reasons to lose weight range from appearance to comfort to health. The amount of weight one wants to drop varies, too. On one end of the spectrum is the person who just wants to drop a couple pounds so her clothes fit better, on the other end are the folks who are morbidly obese who really have to shave off some fat to save their lives.

Most people fall somewhere between these extremes, and our goals vary, too. Some people want to be super lean while others just want to lose some of their excess weight. Recent studies show that losing just 10% of your body weight can improve your health and reduce your risk for diabetes and heart disease. Actress/singer Queen Latifah recently became a spokesperson for a national weight loss program with her goal of losing 10% of her body weight. When she reached her goal she looked great and said she feels great. Is she at her ideal weight according to the BMI (Body Mass Index) charts? No, but she is where she wants to be and is healthy and active.

Doctors will use these BMI charts to determine if you are of "normal" weight, or if you are overweight or obese...or even underweight. The charts are created by a mathematical formula based on a height to weight ratio. They are an improvement from the flat rule of thumb I learned as a teenager that stated at 5'0" you should be 100 lbs and then add 5 pounds for each inch over five feet. Still, I do not believe that we can or should all be neatly compartmentalized into a chart, Latifah is just one example.

Write down your reason(s) for wanting to shed some pounds. You can use the worksheet in the Resources section of this book, or you can go to my website http://www.RefuseToDiet.com/reasons and print one out.

You may have one reason or perhaps several. If you have written down more than one reason put a number by each, ranking them in importance to you.

Now, I want you to categorize your reasons! Next to each reason place the letter A, for appearance, C, for comfort, H, for health or S for should. In my experience all our reasons will fit into one of these categories. Once you are done with that, review your reasons and see if they are complete.

For example, did you write any "A" reasons down? These would be things like "I want to look better", which if you wrote that down it would be very incomplete. Look better for whom? Why is looking better important to you? Will you have more confidence? Be able to connect with people more easily? Will it help you in your work? There is nothing wrong with wanting to look better, but without knowing specifically why you want to look better it really won't be enough of a motivator to keep you going if, when, you face a challenge later.

Similarly, look at any health reasons, like "it is good for me" or "my health will be better" which are also incomplete. How will your health be better? Will you possibly be able to go off medications? Reduce your blood pressure? Take the strain off your knees or back or feet so you experience less pain? Be able to move around more easily and get more fresh air? Avoid a surgery? Safely have a needed surgery?

Drill down to find the complete reasons, the reasons behind the reasons. This is key to your success. That way if you run into a snag on your path, either emotional or physically, it will be much easier to get yourself on track if you know the real reason why you started the journey in the first place.

I want to take a minute to discuss the category "S" reasons. These are things like "My doctor told me I need to," (doctor might be exchanged for mother, husband, wife, or boyfriend) and "I just weigh too much." I call these "should" reasons because they are coming from an external source, not from your own desire. Relook at your ACH reasons now that you have drilled into them. Are any of them "should" reasons? Like, "I should care about my appearance" or "I'm supposed to exercise."

I'm going to go out on a limb here and tell you that until you can honestly own your reasons for losing weight and have them truly be an A, C or H, not an S reason, you will not have success. Oh, you might lose a few pounds, but you will struggle, have more challenges and more than likely put it all back on and more, which we all know is the typical pattern for weight loss.

Louise Hay, author of *You Can Heal Your Life*, states we deserve to eliminate the word "should" from our vocabulary because whenever we use the word "should" we are making ourselves wrong. Either we were wrong, are wrong or will be wrong. I think we've had enough of making ourselves wrong about our weight, so let's focus on health first and comfort and appearance reasons for weight loss.

Look inside yourself for the reasons for improving your health and discover those and you will have a much better chance of achieving the goal and keeping it off. If you are unhappy about your weight or don't feel physically well, there probably is a real reason inside you, even if at first all you are hearing are the "should" messages. Put those messages on the shelf and listen to your inner voice, is it saying "I want to play with my kids without getting out of breath," or "I want to be alive to walk my daughter down the aisle" or some other strong message that deals with yourself and others? If you can't come up with your reason, but you feel strongly that you have one that is not a "should"...you probably do. Take some time to really explore your thoughts and feelings and find that reason. The time you take doing this exercise now will help you in the long run.

As you start your journey to health and fitness and as you continue on the path, keep coming back to your reasons.

Surround Yourself with Love and Positivity

Surround yourself with positive images and experiences. Find experiences that bring you joy and laughter; be in nature, read positive words, meditate, exercise, and give yourself permission to

NOT watch the news. When you surround yourself with love and positivity it is easier to face any challenges that come our way.

"Shower the people you love with love," (from the song by James Taylor)...this includes yourself. You deserve health and happiness and love. By taking care of yourself you will fill your cup up and be able to then shower others with love. If you give all your love away and exhaust yourself, then ultimately you will have no energy for anyone.

How do you talk to yourself? Are you kind and loving to yourself or do you criticize and belittle yourself? Basically emotions come down to two categories: love or fear. If you try to scare, push, threaten or cajole yourself into action you are acting out of fear. A more permanent solution will come if you talk to yourself out of love.

Are you sensitive to what others think? Many of us are "people pleasers" and adapt our desires to what we think others want. We interpret the responses (or lack of response) of others in a way that makes us feel wrong.

Instead, create supportive statements that help you when you recognize other peoples' reactions to any changes you may be experiencing. Unless they honestly tell you what they are thinking, then you are just making up a story. Rather than make up a story that paints you negatively at all, one that tears you down, make up a story that lifts you up and supports you. You don't know what they are thinking, so you be the script writer and you be the star. You get to have all the good lines and all the happy endings!

Loving yourself means not participating in destructive behaviors. That includes overeating or eating foods that cause us ill health. When you love yourself, you take care of yourself, including your body, because it is the right thing to do.

This doesn't mean you are perfect at it—but you will get better and better at it. I have a friend who is a total health food nut. This guy eats only the best organic foods, but he loves ice cream almost as much as I do—even though it makes him physically ill. About once a month or so he will have his ice cream—knowing he will pay for it. His philosophy is to be "good" about 80-90% of the time and that is enough for health.

Loving yourself does not mean that you are not open to improvement. It means that you are done with beating yourself up over the past, because where you are right now is a result of everything you have done in the past and you can't change that.

Loving yourself is choosing to focus on the positive and work on improving yourself bit by bit...now and for the future.

Smile for Weight Loss

Smiling is a great tool for increasing health and weight loss. The act of smiling can actually help you lose weight, not because you burn more calories when you smile (although maybe we do), but because smiling and feeling joyful are great positive aspects of our lives. When we are smiling we are appreciating something in our lives.

I believe that by feeling joy and being grateful for what we have, whether it is that we have the energy and ability to walk in the fresh air, or that we are able to get out of bed today, or whatever little or big thing you can find to be grateful about, we are opening ourselves up to receiving more things to feel grateful about. Including a healthier and more slender body!

This gratitude and happiness helps us to release the emotional bonds that are keeping the fat stuck to us, even if we are "doing everything right". I don't know how else to explain it, but as I said before, the calories in versus calories out model does not always work, so there has to be some other component!

When I am truly appreciating what IS, then I am not worrying about what *might* be or what *was*. I find that I gain weight when I am more focused on the past or the future rather than enjoying the moment. On the other hand, when I am in the present and I am wrapped in that pleasantness...when I allow those feelings to seep into my body I feel a satisfaction that is, well, as good as chocolate slowly melting on my tongue! With a whole lot less calories!

Go do things that trip your "happy button"...things that bring a smile to your face. Make a decision to bring a big smile to your face each and every day. Keep a record of the things that do. Refer to that list when you are feeling blue and use it as a tool to help lift your spirits in those down moments.

Decide that is possible for you to achieve your goals.

At the risk of repeating myself (over and over), affirmations are a great tool to help reinforce this decision.

> "Look in the mirror. Size yourself up.
> Are you the man or woman you want to
> be? If not, give yourself the suggestions
> that can help make you what you desire.
> See a mental picture of how you would
> like to appear to others....Superimpose
> this mental picture upon the actual image
> of yourself before you. See the changes
> you must bring about in yourself, as
> though they had already occurred!
> Repeat this visualization day after day,
> night after night."
>
> Claude Bristol, *TNT The Power Within You*

The mirror is an important tool for a lot of reasons. You recall my dance with the "other woman" at the boutique when I was trying on clothes? That was because I didn't recognize myself. If you don't recognize yourself and believe your new appearance then you will not be able to maintain the change any more than I did.

So you have a choice, learn to recognize yourself as you now are or go back to being who you were. I chose the latter as it turns out. Not consciously of course, but I gained back all my weight so that I was back to being the "big strong girl" I had been. I was back to a size that I could believe and claim, even if I didn't like it, it was what connected up in my brain.

I tried that same diet again and again as my weight spiraled back up. The diet that had been so easy for me that summer was now impossible for me. I believe this was because I was not really ready subconsciously to be slender so I sabotaged my efforts at weight loss. I kept myself safe at a weight that matched my self-image.

The idea is to take your weight drop more slowly and to use the mirror the entire time so you learn to recognize your new body as it changes. Give your brain time to rewire its mental pictures of who you are. Don't label yourself along the way, you don't have to make the images permanently engraved into your brain, you want them to evolve along the way.

It may sound strange when I tell you that you have to learn to recognize yourself as you are right now. We intellectually know we are fat, but most of us don't really see our true selves, how large we really are, any more than the anorexic sees how skinny she has become. How does a person get to be 300 pounds and a size 24 like I was and not really know that she is that big?

I found that our self-image is not founded in reality, we see what we want to see. I allowed myself to get to be 300 pounds because I constantly affirmed that I was fat and ugly and because I only looked at my face in the mirror, and that was just because I washed my face. The face gets fuller gradually and so it was easy to just get used to that. Somehow it was easy to convince myself that I was not "that" fat...I forgot that we don't always really see what the mirror is showing us...our brains and emotions won't always allow us to see the truth. The daily mirror becomes not an accurate representation of who we truly are, but instead a reflection of the person we are willing to admit to being.

If you have ever walked past a storefront and been shocked at the reflection in the glass...that reflection of YOU...then you understand the difference between a true reflection and the daily mirror.

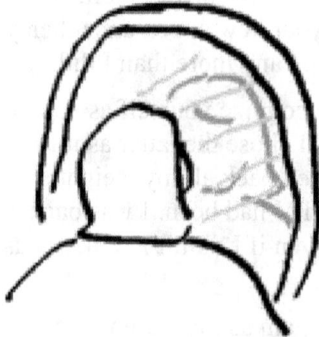

The goal is to now learn to accept our bodies as they are and to get used to the gradual changes that happen as our body gets smaller. That way we recognize ourselves and our brain is not going to try to make us gain weight back to fit the image it holds of us.

To use the mirror for this you have to be able to look at your entire body, or at least most of it. Neck up will not do. Somehow we are completely capable of ignoring the truth of our bellies and thighs when we just look at our faces. My theory on this is that we tend to only look at our eyes, at our soul and our soul is not fat or thin, it just is. By using the mirror we are able to eliminate any cellular confusion that may be going on. We are giving our body, mind and cells time to adjust to the changes that are happening. Think of losing weight like losing a baby blanket. Most of us as children had a blanket or favorite toy that at some point we lost or were forced to give up. We had to adjust to that change; we had to change how we identified ourselves. Suddenly we were a big kid and didn't need that blanket any longer. Well, you have identified with your past size and now you will have to change that. The mirror is where it starts, but it also continues with how you feel. How does it feel different when you get out of bed or the couch or a chair? How is it different when you interact with other people? As long as we recognize that the changes are happening it will be easier to accept that others will notice and other things will feel different. Otherwise we may be confused as to why things are different and try to pull ourselves back so that our experiences match our self-image.

Be loving to yourself when you do this exercise, which you should do every day. Scan your body from head to toe, without judging it good, bad, fat or thin. Just notice where you are and notice changes. The purpose is to cement our self-image in some reality and to also find parts of our physical selves that we can appreciate.

When we feel fat, whether we truly are or not, it is a challenge to be able to look at our bodies with love. Start with a part of your body that you find attractive if you can. If that isn't possible then find a part that you don't hate, or as Abraham says, "start with what you don't loathe" then you can work up to liking and loving.

For me I had to start with my eyes, and even then it was a challenge! But my eyes were the one body part that people would compliment me on. So even if you don't think you are beautiful, can you find something that other people have complimented you on? Start where you can. The idea is to stop focusing on the love handles or thunder thighs and start focusing on positive images.

While you are at the mirror it is also time to practice some supportive, loving affirmations which we have already covered. Use the mirror and loving affirmations to see yourself as you want to be. Look in the mirror and picture yourself in the body you desire with the health that you deserve to have—with that health and happiness shining from your eyes. See yourself and feel it in your heart. Know that this works. I have done it, and you can too!

What Do I Want

How often have you been confused about what exactly you want in your life, but you are positive about what you don't want? We don't want to affirm what we do not want, because we know that only gives us more of it, but sometimes paying a little bit of attention to what we don't want will help guide us to know more clearly what we do want.

A lot of teachers have taught this concept, Michael Losier, author of *Law of Attraction, The Science of Attracting More of What You Want and Less of What You Don't* is one, and he calls the exercise "Clarity through contrast." In *You can Heal Your Life*, Louise Hay teaches pretty much the same thing. We are going to take this exercise and apply it to our bodies and health and thoughts about ourselves.

Take a clean piece of paper and at the top write "What I think about my body" or "my health" or "me". You can use a worksheet from my website to help with this exercise. Go to http://www.RefuseToDiet.com/clarity

Below the header on the left side of the paper write down everything you can think of about your body. Positive thoughts, negative thoughts, loving or hateful thoughts, write them all down. Don't be surprised when you see conflicting thoughts, just write them all down. Don't spend a lot of time doing this and do not edit the list or try to refine it, just quickly write down what comes to mind.

Next take a clean piece of paper and write down only the positive statements that you have from the first list. Rewriting them helps reinforce them in your subconscious.

Identify the first negative thought on the original list and reframe it into a positive, into what you want to be true. In other words, write an affirmation about it. For example, if you wrote, "I hate my fat thighs," one way to change that might be to write "My thighs get thinner every day because I am making healthy choices," or you might say "My legs are strong and sturdy and carry me easily from place to place." Find something that speaks to you.

By shining a little light on the negative thoughts, we are bringing them to the surface. By revealing them we can begin to change them. This can be a painful or scary process, I know. I didn't want to face these thoughts and for a long time I didn't think I had to. Somehow I imagined that by bringing them up it would either unleash a monster or lead to my blaming someone else for my situation. My intellect said, "They did the best they could" and it felt safer to keep my "inner monster" corked up. However it wasn't until I let it out that I made real progress and was able to, once and for all, lose weight.

It isn't about blaming other people; it isn't about blaming yourself. It is about taking emotions and thoughts that may not even be based in any kind of reality and bringing them to the light of day so you can face them and change them, and change your life into the one you want it to be.

During this process you may find that you have to forgive yourself. If your list has a lot of negative comments about you as a person, then you may choose to turn those into "I forgive myself" statements.

- I forgive myself for all the hurts I have caused myself and others
- I forgive myself for all the times I acted in ways I am less than proud of
- I am a loveable and loving human being
- I love myself just the way I am

Here are some other examples of negative thoughts, and how they may be turned around.

- "I am fat" becomes "I am on the path to having a healthy slender body"
- "I am ugly" becomes "My inner beauty shines through for the world to see"
- "I am grotesque" becomes "I am a beloved child of God"
- "No one could love this body" becomes "My body is the temple that houses my spirit, and people see my spirit and love me"

If nothing comes up when you do this exercise then it might not be the right time for you. Not very many people truly can say they have no negative thoughts about themselves or their body. Don't force it—just come back to it another time. It is also possible that this topic may not be right for you, but since you are reading this book about losing weight, improving your body, then I suspect there are at least one or two negative thoughts hiding in your subconscious. If there were none, then it should be an easy matter for you to drop weight, and you probably wouldn't have a lot of excess pounds to start with. But sometimes we aren't aware of the negative thinking that is holding us back. So, again, if nothing comes up for you right now, give yourself permission to come back to this later. Just let the idea "steep" for a bit. That may be all it takes for your conscious mind to then recognize any negative thoughts when they do come up.

On the other hand, if you find some super strong emotions come up, or thoughts scare you, then consider working with a professional therapist. If at any time you have serious thoughts of harming yourself or someone else, consult a professional. Remember, I am not a doctor, I was an art major, okay?

Once you have identified what you don't want, and then have turned it around to what you do want, don't read them over; don't repeat them. Shred the paper with the negative thoughts. You only want to keep the new sheet that is filled with positive thoughts.

Now that you are aware of those thoughts it may be easier for you to stop the negative thoughts by practicing a "pattern interrupt"...I include a tool on that in Chapter 8. For now, focus on the positive thoughts!

Tools: pleasure log, gratitude journal, celebrating results

Remember when you got gold stars in school, or badges in scouts? I am suggesting that you give yourself some gold stars every day. For some of you, the thought of that just made you very uncomfortable. If it did, then perhaps, like me, you struggle with the idea that we have to be perfect to deserve the badge.

When I think back to Girl Scouts and getting those badges, I realize that getting the badge didn't mean I had mastered the task. It meant that I had learned something new. Keep on learning and applying yourself, and taking credit for that learning. Every night write down five things you did that day that deserve to be recognized, celebrated or that you are grateful for. I know some nights I have to search pretty hard to get five down! But by remembering the positive things I did that day, whether it was making a healthy food choice, taking a flight of stairs, doing something nice for someone else, or even accepting a compliment graciously, we are training our brains to remember the good things in our lives. We are planting seeds that reinforce we are good and loving and worthy people. Every time we do that, it will be easier to remember the good things the next day.

Remembering your good "stuff" helps you to recognize that you are good, and that you are worthy. So the tool is to keep a journal; it doesn't have to be fancy or filled with lots of writing. It can be a traditional journal, or just a series of lists, but every night write down five positive statements about yourself or what you accomplished that day. They don't have to be health or fitness related, they certainly can be, but don't limit yourself. Look at your entire day and life, because that is what Refuse to Diet is all about, your entire life!

Another thing to write in your journal is notes on other people who inspire you. This isn't about competition, and it doesn't have to be about their weight loss. You don't have to write reams about it, just jot down what you notice and how you felt about it. Sometimes someone will inspire you with their attitude or that they have a certain energy, or maybe they showed you a new exercise or healthy eating choice. It might be that just their success is an inspiration because it demonstrates to you that it is possible to gain health.

Review the notes you make in this journal periodically. You will be amazed to see how much you have grown to be a wonderful composite of all the traits you admired in others.

Awaken with Gratitude

"As each day comes to us refreshed and anew, so does my gratitude renew itself daily. The breaking of the sun over the horizon is my grateful heart dawning upon a blessed world."

~Adabella Radici

Feeding your mind and soul with thoughts of gratitude before you fall asleep is an excellent practice. It is also a great habit to get into in the morning. If you watched the movie, "The Secret" you saw it mentioned there. Many teachers suggest you run through a list of things for which you feel gratitude as you rise and get out of bed in the morning.

A friend of mine told me she was having trouble thinking of things to be grateful for. I know this can be a challenge when you are going through a rough spell—the exact time we need it the most! When I am feeling down, I have some very simple, basic things I remember I am grateful for. *Nothing* is too small to express your gratitude.

- I am grateful for the sight that I have
- I am grateful for my strong legs, and the feet that carry me through the day
- I am grateful that I can smell the flowers in the garden
- I am grateful I can hear the birds singing outside
- I am grateful that I am safe with a roof over my head

By appreciating these things we open ourselves up for even more things to be grateful for!

"If you want to turn your life around, try thankfulness. It will change your life mightily."

~Gerald Good

Chapter 6: Measuring Weight Loss Success

"Judging your weight loss success on the scale is like driving forward while looking in the rearview mirror."

~Laurie Tossy

Objective Numbers

I'm not really fond of using numbers too much for gauging our success, but I do believe they can be useful tools because they are objective. They aren't subject to our emotions, to interpretations, to being washed and shrunk, or worn and stretched out. They just are.

Realize that your current size and weight is a reflection of things you did and choices you made in the past. There is no benefit to beating yourself up over it. Just let them be objective numbers. Judging your success on the scale is like driving forward while looking in the rearview mirror. You are going in two different directions. Set the state for your future by focusing on what you are doing now, rather than focusing on the past by fixating on the scale. To get an accurate view of the road ahead you must look forward through the windshield.

That being said, people love to measure themselves. I know that, and it can be very satisfying to say "I have lost over 120 pounds." So, if you choose to use numbers as a tool, then I suggest you use a lot of numbers. Don't just rely on the scale, because that only gives you partial information. Take your measurements-- especially your waist, hips, upper arms and thighs. Also I prefer a scale that includes body fat percentage. They aren't 100% accurate, but you can get a decent one for home use which doesn't cost too much money. The reason I suggest them is when you are exercising you will be increasing your muscles and you have probably heard that muscle weighs more than fat. By using a scale that registers both weight and body fat, you can actually prove to yourself that your health routine is working—even if the weight number hasn't moved. It is a great tool to help keep your attitude up when you hit a plateau.

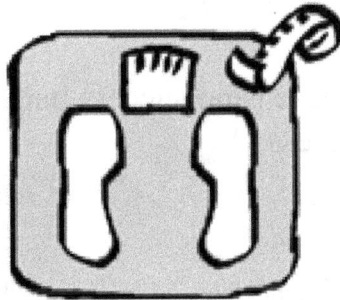

There is a danger in using scales though. If you don't focus on your mindset first, then the scale can become an extremely powerful and dangerous tool to defeat you. It is very easy to place too much weight, as it were, on the number on the scale.

I once was as addicted to the number on the scale as I was to food, often getting on the scale three or more times in a day. That's not counting the times I got on and off it right in a row, moving the scale a few inches trying to find the "sweet spot" on the bathroom floor.

So if you choose to weigh yourself, I suggest you do so no more frequently that once a week. Anything more often than that doesn't accurately reflect real weight loss, and can be demoralizing or lead to false conclusions about what does, or does not work for us.

Most people have a general idea about how much they "should" weigh, or how much they want to weigh. Your doctor may have a different number in mind for you.

Most doctors will simply refer to the BMI, so it can be helpful to know where you "should" fall on that index. For that reason, I have included a copy of the BMI (Body Mass Index) chart for your reference. Use it as a guide, but don't stress about getting to an exact number. If you have large bones and are athletic with a lot of muscle, you will weigh more than the chart indicates you "should." And if you feel physically and emotionally better with a few pounds more than the chart dictates, listen to your body. Your body is a lot smarter than any chart. Remember Queen Latifah and go for health and what feels good, not a number.

"There is no success but your own success."

~Leslie Grimutter

Supplement the numbers on the scale with monthly measurements. Keep a record of your measurements so you can see your progress.

Body Mass Index (BMI) Chart

Obese BMI>30   Overweight BMI 25-30   Normal BMI 18.5-25   Underweight BMI <18.5

HEIGHT in feet/inches

WEIGHT in lbs	4'8"	4'9"	4'10"	4'11"	5'0"	5'1"	5'2"	5'3"	5'4"	5'5"	5'6"	5'7"	5'8"	5'9"	5'10"	5'11"	6'0"	6'1"	6'2"	6'3"	6'4"	6'5"
260	58	56	54	53	51	49	48	46	45	43	42	41	40	38	37	36	35	34	33	32	32	31
255	57	55	53	51	50	48	47	45	44	42	41	40	39	38	37	36	35	34	33	32	31	30
250	56	54	52	50	49	47	46	44	43	42	40	39	38	37	36	35	34	33	32	31	30	30
245	55	53	51	49	48	46	45	43	42	41	40	38	37	36	35	34	33	32	31	31	30	29
240	54	52	50	48	47	45	44	43	41	40	39	38	36	35	34	33	33	32	31	30	29	28
235	53	51	49	47	46	44	43	42	40	39	38	37	36	35	34	33	32	31	30	29	29	28
230	52	50	48	46	45	43	42	41	39	38	37	36	35	34	33	32	31	30	30	29	28	27
225	50	49	47	45	44	43	41	40	39	37	36	35	34	33	32	31	31	30	29	28	27	27
220	49	48	46	44	43	42	40	39	38	37	36	34	33	32	32	31	30	29	28	27	27	26
215	48	47	45	43	42	41	39	38	37	36	35	34	33	32	31	30	29	28	28	27	26	25
210	47	45	44	42	41	40	38	37	36	35	34	33	32	31	30	29	28	28	27	26	26	25
205	46	44	43	41	40	39	38	37	36	35	34	33	32	31	30	29	28	27	26	26	25	24
200	45	43	42	40	39	38	37	35	34	33	32	31	30	30	29	28	27	26	26	25	24	24
195	44	42	41	39	38	37	36	35	33	32	31	31	30	29	28	27	26	26	25	24	24	23
190	43	41	40	38	37	36	35	34	33	32	31	30	29	28	27	26	26	25	24	24	23	23
185	41	40	39	37	36	35	34	33	32	31	30	29	28	27	27	26	25	24	24	23	23	22
180	40	39	38	36	35	34	33	32	31	30	29	28	27	27	26	25	24	24	23	22	22	21
175	39	38	37	35	34	33	32	31	30	29	28	27	27	26	25	24	24	23	22	22	21	21
170	38	37	36	34	33	32	31	30	29	28	27	27	26	25	24	24	23	22	22	21	21	20
165	37	36	34	33	32	31	30	29	28	27	27	26	25	24	24	23	22	22	21	21	20	20
160	36	35	33	32	31	30	29	28	27	27	26	25	24	24	23	22	22	21	21	20	19	19
155	35	34	32	31	30	29	28	27	27	26	25	24	24	23	22	22	21	20	20	19	19	18
150	34	32	31	30	29	28	27	27	26	25	24	23	23	22	22	21	20	20	19	19	18	18
145	33	31	30	29	28	27	27	26	25	24	23	23	22	21	21	20	20	19	19	18	18	17
140	31	30	29	28	27	26	26	25	24	23	23	22	21	21	20	20	19	18	18	17	17	17
135	30	29	28	27	26	26	25	24	23	22	22	21	21	20	19	19	18	18	17	17	16	16
130	29	28	27	26	25	25	24	23	22	22	21	20	20	19	19	18	18	17	17	16	16	15
125	28	27	26	25	24	24	23	22	21	21	20	20	19	18	18	17	17	16	16	16	15	15
120	27	26	25	24	23	23	22	21	21	20	19	19	18	18	17	17	16	16	15	15	15	14
115	26	25	24	23	22	22	21	20	20	19	19	18	17	17	16	16	16	15	15	14	14	14
110	25	24	23	22	21	21	20	19	19	18	18	17	17	16	16	15	15	15	14	14	13	13
105	24	23	22	21	21	20	19	19	18	18	17	17	16	16	15	15	14	14	13	13	13	12
100	22	22	21	20	20	19	18	18	17	17	16	16	15	15	14	14	14	13	13	12	12	12
95	21	21	20	19	19	18	17	17	16	16	15	15	14	14	14	13	13	13	12	12	12	11
90	20	19	19	18	18	17	16	16	15	15	15	14	14	13	13	13	12	12	12	11	11	11
85	19	18	18	17	17	16	16	15	15	14	14	13	13	13	12	12	12	11	11	11	10	10
80	18	17	17	16	16	15	15	14	14	13	13	13	12	12	11	11	11	11	10	10	10	9

Note: BMI values are rounded to nearest whole number.

BMI categories are based on Centers for Disease Control and Prevention criteria.

Other Measures of Success

Notice and celebrate other measures of weight loss success, too. They may be less "objective," but that doesn't make them less valid, or valuable!

Do you feel your clothes getting looser? Are you fitting into your "skinny" clothes? Are all your clothes too big? How about your bra...you're apt to need a new one, ladies!

You may actually be surprised at some of the things you notice...if you drop a significant amount of weight even your shoes will become big! I have a necklace that I thought was tiny—I can wear it now comfortably, and I can't stand anything tight on my neck!

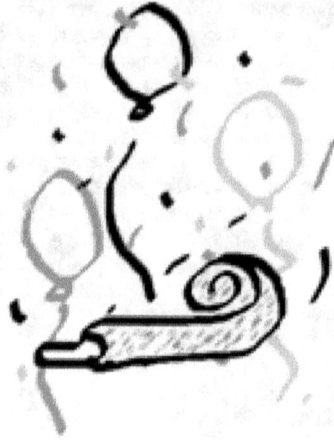

Do you have trouble buckling your seatbelt? Do you need seatbelt extensions? Notice and appreciate when that gets easier, and the extensions are no longer necessary!

When at the doctor's office, does the nurse have to go to a different room to get a blood pressure cuff that fits? One of my big "Wow!" moments was when I was donating blood, and for the first time they didn't have to get the extra large cuff. When suddenly that's not needed any more—that's a big accomplishment.

Notice your fitness level, too. Can you walk further? Faster? Is it easier to catch your breath? Do you get out of breath less often? I notice that walking is so much easier now...and I am less concerned that I might hurt myself...my knees are more stable.

These are all wonderful measures of success. Acknowledge them and celebrate them!

Other Numbers

The next time you have blood work done, get a copy of all your numbers. Track your cholesterol, blood sugar levels, etc. See how these numbers change as you improve your health, drop excess fat and move around more.

If you need help interpreting your numbers, seeing how they are improving, ask your doctor, or you can consult with another practitioner.

My mother recently had blood work done and was unclear on what some of her numbers meant. The test results were mailed to her, rather than being given to her during an appointment with a doctor, so she made a phone appointment with my friend, Dr. Linda Larson. Dr. Linda is a Ph.D. prepared Family Nurse Practitioner. Her specialty is endocrinology...and she has a broad base of knowledge from nearly 40 years of practicing medicine. Dr. Linda reviewed all the numbers with my mom, and helped guide her on questions to ask her primary care physician later. If that sounds like something that would be helpful to you, check the resources section in the back where you can see how to schedule a consult with Dr. Linda.

Bottom line—don't rely on just one number. Your life is much more than a single number! Look at the entire picture—the numbers, how you look and most importantly <u>how you feel</u>. That full picture is a much better measure of success than just a number on the scale!

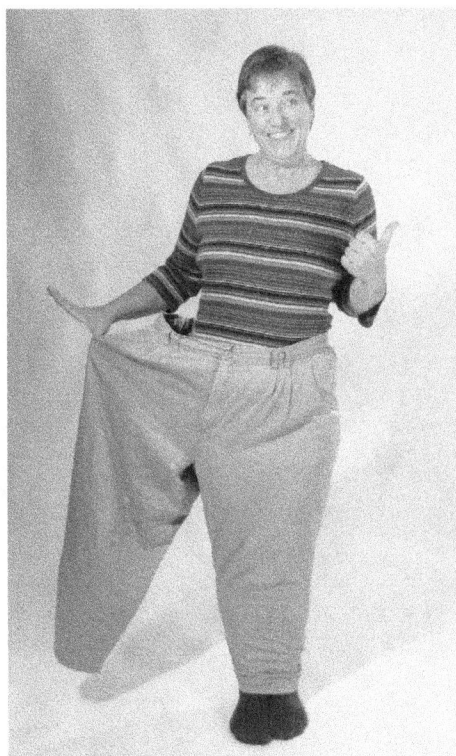

Chapter 7: Getting Real—Where You Are and Where You Are Going

> "How can you know where you are going if you don't know where you are starting from?"
>
> ~Laurie Tossy

Challenges We Face

Everyone who has ever tried to lose weight, whether it is a couple pounds or more than 100, knows there are challenges. If it were easy, there wouldn't be a problem!

Some of the typical challenges faced are

- Not liking to exercise

- Craving carbohydrates (sugars, breads, pastas, etc)

- Lack of time—to exercise, to prepare healthy meals, to eat foods that are good for you

- Having to fix meals for others and not wanting to prepare different foods for yourself

- Traveling for business or pleasure

- Believing you lack self-discipline or willpower

- Hating to fail

- Physical limitations due to pain or body size

- Feeling self-conscious

- Emotional attachment to food, emotional eating

At least one of these challenges is typically faced by anyone who wants to drop a few pounds. If you are obese, chances are you are faced with several of them, and the emotions attached to the challenges are probably larger.

So what can you do to beat the challenges, and win the weight loss game—in a manner that is healthy and permanent?

First, realize you are not alone. We are facing an epidemic of obesity.

Next, look beyond those people and find evidence that people have successfully lost weight. Ask yourself, "Do I know anyone who has lost weight? Have I read a single article or headline about someone having lost weight?" Know that you are just as capable as they are, and if ANYONE, ANYWHERE has ever lost weight, then you can, too!

Make a commitment to your health. By placing the focus on your health, as opposed to a number on the scale, you are encouraging changes that will be permanent versus a "diet" which is by nature, short-term.

Claim your health goal. Be realistic and health focused, rather than saying "I am going to lose 20 pounds by Sue's wedding next month," say "I am taking control of my life by making healthy food choices and moving my body more every day." Simply claiming it will help bring you positive results.

I have a friend who has committed to become a doctor. She has chosen the path, and is moving forward on that path every day. She has lots to learn and practice, and she knows she will face challenges along the way. She is going to take them one at a time, because that is all part of getting from where she is now to where she wants to be. Every exam she takes, every hour of residency brings her closer. If she quit at any point she wouldn't reach her goal.

Your goal has to be as strong. Like her, you will face challenges and set-back—and like her, if you quit you'll never reach your goal. And also like her, every moment moves you closer to that goal.

The Blame Game

Accept personal responsibility. For what you weigh now and for every decision you make regarding food and exercise. Don't beat yourself up over them, but recognize that it was your choices that got you where you are—and it will be your choices that will get you back to health, too! As long as you blame others or shame yourself, you will not be able to achieve a healthy weight permanently.

I definitely loved playing the blame game. I wanted to blame anyone and everyone rather than take responsibility for my weight. It was my mother's fault, then my doctor's, then my ex's. I blamed my job, stress, my bone structure, my genes, society, our dependence on the automobile. You name it, I blamed it! I finally realized there was one culprit who was present each and every time I got fat, every time I didn't work out, every time I over ate, every time I came up with an excuse, whether justified or far-fetched. I finally found the one place where blame could rightfully rest. I faced the enemy, and saw that it was ME.

Your Mouth Is Not the Problem

For years I bought into the idea that my mouth was what got me into trouble. I even started to "blame" my mouth, saying I had an oral fixation. I saw cigarette smokers as having a similar problem, but an easier time, in a way. Like alcoholics and drug addicts, smokers can choose to never smoke again. You can't do that with food. You have to eat to live; you can't just quit eating and expect to survive. Slowly I realized that I was a drug addict, and that my drug of choice was food.

I'm serious about referring to food as my drug of choice. The truth is, whether we use prescriptions, street drugs, alcohol or food, we are drugging ourselves. We are numbing ourselves. That is a critical thing we have to realize. Now, if you are a few pounds overweight then this may not be your issue, but if you have struggled your entire life to be a healthy weight, or if you are more than "a little bit" overweight, then there are some bigger issues at play.

Using food as a drug is acceptable in our society. People aren't fired for eating donuts—in fact bosses will frequently bring them in as rewards! You probably haven't lost your house because of food, or killed anybody because you were driving while on a sugar "high." Food addiction allows us to maintain a modicum of control. We can numb ourselves in a safer, more socially acceptable manner, to a point. Even when we are obese, and it is no longer socially acceptable, we are viewed differently from other addicts. Obese people are generally looked upon as lazy or not caring. Because we don't poison others with second-hand smoke or endanger people's lives when we drive, we aren't shunned in quite the same way. We aren't forced to have our coffee breaks outside in the rain and snow. This also allows us to put on a "holier-than-thou" suit, when really we are the same inside, a mere mortal dealing with an addiction.

I looked at my body with disgust and wondered how could I do that to myself? I wondered if people looked at me and asked themselves, "How much food does she have to eat to get to be that big?"

The truth was, it didn't actually take a lot of food, and I mostly ate a healthy diet. I knew what to eat, and generally made healthy choices. Of course I had my weaknesses, but even "good" food when eaten in large quantities will be enough to keep you fat. Doctors will claim it is a simple matter of physics: you have to take in fewer calories than you spend, so if you are over fat you must either reduce your intake or increase the out go. Simple. HA! I found it was far from simple—and I'll bet you have, too.

If my mouth was truly the source of the problem, then it stands to reason my mouth would have been the solution. Diets would work if our mouths were the problem. Having tried dozens and dozens of them, and still managing to be fat, I had proof that my weight issue was not going to be resolved by dieting and my mouth.

There are some basics to nutrition that we need to know, but really...do you believe a cup of ice cream is a healthy choice for daily dairy servings?, that fried okra counts as a vegetable?, that a "pat" of butter is ¼ of a stick?, or a "serving" of bread is half a loaf? If you do, then you deserve to get to the library or bookstore and get a couple books on nutrition, or set up an appointment with a nutritionist or diet coach, because you need those basic building blocks to create a healthy body. If you already know the basics and are having trouble with making those choices, with living a healthy life, and would like to put an end to the struggle once and for all, then keep on reading.

Small and Consistent is Key

"Success will never be a big step in the future, success is a small step taken just now."

~Jonaton Mårtensson

Start small and be consistent. Add 5-10 minutes of moving your body more. Exchange one unhealthy eating habit for a better one. Keep with it and over time you will lose weight. Every week make another small change. Soon you will be amazed at how different you feel and look—and you will have incorporated these new habits into your life!

Get support—reach out to someone who is in the same boat, and you can buoy each other during the journey! Support and accountability are awesome ways to get through the hurdles that will come up.

Know that there will be setbacks and obstacles along the way, so have a plan on how to deal with them. Refer to the Options list you created; add to it when you come up with new ideas! How will you handle the food at the office party? How will you plan ahead for the upcoming business trip? What measures can you take to reduce emotional eating? What can my family members do to help me to achieve my goal? The true failure is never starting…or not getting back up when you fall. This is for your LIFE, not a week or a month, so just keep plugging away

We are human and therefore aren't "perfect" (as much as we might like to be.) This is true in all of our behaviors—including our health and fitness goals.

Even with the best intentions, it is easy to stray from our chosen path if we don't pay attention and be present.

One of my personal challenges is allowing myself to get so busy that I don't take ample breaks…or I will work until late in the evening. I will "forget" to meditate or to eat….or even just to get up and move.

In the very short-term, these added moments seem like they move me forward. I spend more time at a project so I get it done faster…I don't eat, so I must be taking in fewer calories, so I must lose weight.

Truth is, these patterns ultimately set me back—by causing greater fatigue, disharmony and even weight gain. Instead of pacing myself and taking care of my body, I will push and push and push. If I don't stop myself I will push until I break. Then, on one extreme I might get physically ill. On the other hand it may be that I "just" discover that I'm famished and so I eat, and eat and eat. By not eating for long periods of time I set myself up to binge eat later…my blood sugar levels are out of whack and my moods are erratic.

I am far better off taking breaks, eating on a regular basis, doing all the things that I know to do to stay healthy: eat, sleep, move my body, play, and work.

Rather than beat myself up over it, my goal is to be loving and gentle and guide myself firmly, and lovingly back to the path that I know works for me.

This gives me the opportunity to recognize how my body feels and to evaluate that. Have I been paying attention? I also have the chance to reflect on my behaviors. Have I picked up some new "bad" habits…or perhaps slipped into an old familiar pattern that is not in my best health interests?

The reason to look at any less healthy choices I may have been making is so I can stop or modify them and replace them with healthier ones—not to flog myself for my "mistakes." Those actions were in the past (even if it was only yesterday, or even just an hour ago!)

It is up to me to see how I can do better—NOW and in the future.

I choose to proclaim what I have done RIGHT and focus on continuing those behaviors and improving those positive skills!

Make Small Changes

> "If nothing ever changed, there'd be no butterflies."
>
> ~Author Unknown

Don't try to change everything all at once. Again, make small changes; get that change into your new health pattern, then make another small change. To do this, it is helpful to have a realistic idea about what you are doing now. It is so easy to fool ourselves. We ingest calories without even being aware, because of our habits and unconscious eating.

Assess Your Current Situation

In business we set benchmarks. We establish what our current situation or benchmark is so we can identify areas to improve, and to later evaluate our progress. That is what I suggest you do.

Be objective: pretend you are a scientist studying the habits of an animal in the wild. The scientist doesn't criticize the animal for what it does or doesn't do. They just record the data. Put on your objective scientist hat and record what you do.

The goal is to get to know yourself, and to discover what your biggest challenges are. Are you pressed for time? Do you rely on sugar or caffeine for energy? Do you hate to cook? Do you have physical limitations that keep you from doing any kind of exercise?

I contend that our biggest challenge comes from our mindset, our belief in our ability to attain health; belief that we are worthy of health. This is what self-love is. Self-love has gotten a bad rap in a lot of places; it has been misconstrued as being egotistical, stuck-up, selfish, narcissistic; that is not what I'm talking about.

Think about someone you love, it could be a child, a parent, a friend, a partner or even a pet. Now think about what you want for them. What did you come up with? Health? Love? Financial freedom? A good job? Safety?

Is it bad for you to want these things for them? Are you depriving anyone else of good because you want these things for your loved one? Of course not! So if it is not bad to want these things for someone else, and you are not depriving others by wanting these things for someone else, then why is it wrong to want them for yourself? It isn't! This is the kind of self-love that I'm talking about, a love that wants the best possible life for you. To love yourself enough to want what is in your best interest, to know you deserve it, and to take the action steps to achieve it.

Establishing Your BenchMark

1. **Get a journal to write in.**

   It could be a notebook like you used in school or a hardbound journal. It doesn't really matter what you use as long as it will work for you. I suggest it be small enough you can carry it with you easily in your purse, pocket or briefcase. If you use a day planner, you can incorporate it into that system. If you use a PDA, you can have your journal there. The point is you don't have to spend a lot of money on this, or a lot of time figuring out a system. If you have a system that works for your calendar and appointments, as long as it is portable, use that. Otherwise pick up a little notebook at the grocery store and you are good to go.

   You will be recording data for one week. It will be tempting to modify your eating or drinking during this time, but do your best not to. This is about establishing where you truly are right now so you can see where to go. No one but you will see this unless you choose to share it. It is not being "turned in"; you are not being "graded." It is not about being right or wrong, good or bad.

   Let's face it, you wouldn't be reading this book if you didn't have some concerns about your weight. You are simply going to identify the truth, without judging it, so you can clearly see what is working for you, and what is not.

2. **Drink**

   Write down every drink you take, including water, for this week. Don't worry if there is a party or special event, just write down what you drink. There is always some event that we can use as an excuse to overindulge, so be real about it, and if it comes up during this week that is okay.

Know how many ounces you are drinking if at all possible. Frequently we think we are drinking more water than we really are because we don't count how many glasses we drink. On the other hand, we tend to underestimate how much we consume of other drinks, such as soda, fruit juice, milk and alcohol, because we don't really know how many ounces our glass or mug holds.

I realize if you are at someone else's home, or at a party, or a restaurant, you might not be able to know the ounces in the glass. But for your own glasses and mugs at home and work you can measure how many ounces they hold and write that in your journal. That way you can write, "10 oz coffee, black" or "16 oz coffee with cream and sugar" or "18 oz diet soda," etc.

If you don't know how many ounces your favorite glass or mug holds, here's a simple way to measure it. Have a large measuring cup with lines indicating the ounces on it. I find clear glass is the easiest to use—but use what you have. If possible, it should hold at least two cups of liquid.

Fill your favorite mug with water. Pour the water from the mug into the measuring cup. Now at the beginning of your journal write a description of the mug and how many ounces it holds.

Repeat this process for every size glass that you use regularly. If you use a giant mug, you might have to refill your measuring cup more than once and add the ounces together to get your total, but for most standard household glassware a two cup measurer will be sufficient to get it in one pass.

3. **Food**

   Just like with your drinks, write down every bite that you eat this week.

   Rather than weighing everything in ounces I suggest you write in approximate dimensions or relative terms. For example, you can write, hunk of cheese about 1x3".

   Write from your personal experience about sizes. Did you have one scoop of ice cream, or did you have a large bowl or half gallon?

   Be sure to write down if you went for seconds or thirds.

Did you have any vegetables? What kind? Did they have a sauce? Were they fried?

One note about measuring food, it is helpful to know the quantities you eat but if that is going to keep you from writing things down then just write down what you ate. The idea is not to make this a chore; you are looking for the starting line so you have a more accurate perception of the course ahead.

4. Feelings

For a lot of people this is the hardest part, but it is also one of the most important and eye-opening sections.

Write down any feelings that come up before, during and after eating. Later you'll use this feeling section to help identify triggers that you have.

Example: "I saw a plate full of donuts at work but didn't have any because I didn't want people to see the fat girl eating. But I kept thinking about those donuts. Later at lunch I ate a big plate of food but still felt hungry. Then I really overdid it at dinner. How am I going to ever lose weight?"

Or, "had a fight with my husband. He really ticked me off. He doesn't understand how hard I am working."

"The kids were so loud today it really grated on my nerves."

"I had a great day today I felt so happy. I feel like celebrating, my boss told me I am doing a great job."

"I feel tired, I'm physically drained. I didn't sleep well."

Remember to be that objective scientist. Don't judge the emotion; they are not good or bad; simply record them. Your goal is to later make some permanent changes to improve your health. It is crucial to know where you are now in order to make those changes.

5. Movement

Record how often you moved your body, whether it is "official" exercise, walking to get the mail, or vacuuming...it all counts!

If you have a pedometer—then get it out. If you don't have one and you can swing about $15-20 you might want to get one. Set it up according to the instructions. It is easy and only takes a few minutes. This will allow the pedometer to count the number of steps you take in a day. At the end of the day write in your journal the number of steps you took.

If you don't have a pedometer then you can write things like "I walked from my car to the office," and "I walked up and down the stairs three times while cleaning the house."

Once that week has passed you are done collecting data. You recorded what you ate, drank, how you felt and how much you moved your body. Good job!

The next step is to analyze the data. Don't let this stress you out, and don't think you have to do it in one sitting.

Look at the entire week and average how many ounces you drank of water and other beverages. Don't add all the beverages together though. Take each one separately.

For example, you might note something like this

On average I drank two 8 ounce glasses of water a day, six 12 oz cans of diet soda and four 10oz cups of coffee

Look at the movement you made during the week. If you had a pedometer how many steps did you take on average? Less than 1000? More than 5000?

A lot of people will see a pattern that is really different between work days and weekend, or non-work, days. It might be that you move significantly more on days that you work, or perhaps you move a lot less. Same with food and drink. If you see significant differences between your food or drink intake, how much moving you do, or your emotions, that is really good to know. In that case, it would be helpful to have two separate benchmarks, one for workdays and one for weekends.

Now take your measurements. These are the "objective numbers" that will help you to see your progress later; your measure of success as we covered in Chapter 6. Measure your weight, your inches, note the clothing sizes you wear. I also suggest you take a photo of yourself as a reference...you can refer to the photo tool in Chapter 5.

When you look at what you consumed during the week, search for patterns. Do you always have a soda in the middle of the afternoon? Do you eat the same foods on a regular basis? Do you eat a lot of simple sugars (white bread, sweets, pasta)? Do you eat a large amount of any particular food—burgers, fries, ice cream, bread and butter, meat, diet drinks? Do you eat a fairly balanced diet, but large portions of everything? Write down anything that jumps out at you as you read the journal, especially if it surprises you.

Looking at your moods and feelings, see you if you notice any patterns between your feelings and how much, or what, you ate or drank, and write those observations down.

For example, "I ate ice cream whenever I felt sad or worried," or "I noticed that when I felt mad I ate salty foods," or "I noticed that when I overeat I always beat myself up afterwards," or "When I felt stressed I ate anything and everything," or "I noticed that when I told myself I shouldn't eat something I ended up eating more later in the day."

Now that you have analyzed the data and identified your patterns, it is time for you to decide what small change you are going to make in the area of movement and food/drink consumption to improve your health.

Set some super easy to achieve goals for the next week. I suggest they be things you absolutely know you can do. It takes three weeks to change habits, and that is what you are doing, so make it something that you can make a sacred commitment to yourself to keeping.

By making small steps, you will keep that commitment. This allows your subconscious to start to believe you when you tell it you will follow through. After all, how many times have you said you would exercise more, eat less, do this diet, lose x pounds, etc... and how many times did you break that promise to yourself?

Believe me, there is a part of you that does not believe it when you say you are going to do this; that you are really serious this time. You may even hear that little voice saying "Yeah, right, I've heard that before," "Oh sure you will, what makes this time any different?" or "You can't lose weight, you are a worthless slob, just give up now so you don't humiliate yourself by failing yet again."

Don't listen to that voice, to those negative messages. Instead, start to change them by making small changes in your life, committing to small changes and actually following through. That is what will stop those inner critics!

So if you average 3000 steps a day, set your promise at 3300 a day not 6000. A 10% increase is very doable. If you didn't move at all, set a goal to move for five minutes. If you don't have a pedometer than use a time or visual distance goal such as "I will walk to the end of the block." Just make it something that you can say "Yes, I did it!"

Make a promise to yourself specifically about how much water you will drink. It might be that you add one 8 ounce glass of water a day.

Remember...my philosophy is that I refuse to diet, but that doesn't mean I won't be changing my eating habits. You started with learning to change your mind and to care for your health and body. That alone is going to help you improve your eating habits, but you can also use your journal to identify times when you tended to eat without realizing it, or ate a lot more than you really realized.

Look for the "low lying fruit" when you review your journal. That is the places that really surprised you, along with the empty calories. If you are drinking sodas or alcohol regularly, you can cut back there and save a couple hundred calories. Don't make any huge changes all at once; this isn't about deprivation. Make some small changes and let them be permanent.

Write in your journal the promises you are making to yourself, and every day write down how you did at keeping that promise.

Every week you can repeat this process. If you found you didn't meet your commitment to yourself, then make the new commitment smaller. If you did succeed at keeping to your commitment, then you can make another small change to your activity or what you are ingesting. Once you have fulfilled your promise to yourself then you are building a foundation of truth: truth that you can follow through, and truth that you can take the steps and make changes.

The main purpose of this journal is to get to know yourself, how you spend your day, and what your biggest food challenges are.

Getting to Know You

One of the things that you will want to keep in mind is we are all different. We all have different food challenges, as well as other challenges, that affect our weight and health.

In your journal, write down what your biggest food challenges are. Here are some things you can consider:

- Are you pressed for time and therefore eat a lot of takeout?

- Do you eat a lot of sugar for the energy boost?

- Is food an emotional release for you?

- Is food your best friend?

- Do you love to cook? Or hate to cook?

- Do you eat breakfast? Is it on the run?

- Do you eat lunch and dinner?

- Do you snack through the day?

- Do you like to eat late at night?

- How much time do you realistically have for meal prep?

- Do you have others that you prepare meals for? Other adults? Kids?

- Do you or they have any dietary restrictions?

Other potential challenges:
- Do you hate to exercise?

- Do you have low energy and think you don't have energy to exercise?

- Do you not have the space or a place to exercise?

- Are you embarrassed about your body and don't want people to see you working out?

- Are you concerned you don't know what to do, where to start?

- Do you have physical limitations that might restrict your ability to exercise?

Everyone has challenges that they face. What may be a big challenge for me may seem like nothing at all to you. And what seems insurmountable to you might seem like a breeze to your spouse, co-worker or best friend. The important thing is to be aware of what challenges YOU have, so that you can know where you are right now, because how can you know where you are going if you don't know where you are starting from?

We'll cover more challenges and how to deal with them in the following chapters. We'll talk about challenges with exercise specifically in Chapter 12.

Chapter 8: Emotional and Unconscious Eating

"It's not so much that we're afraid of
change or so in love with the old
ways, but it's that place in between
that we fear... .It's like being between
trapezes. It's Linus when his blanket
is in the dryer. There's nothing to
hold on to."

~Marilyn Ferguson

Emotional Eating

We covered some emotions earlier in Chapter 5, but it is such a big reason why so many of us overeat and hold onto our body fat it deserves some more attention.

Be aware that emotions will come up along the way. One of the biggest emotions people face when it comes to losing weight is fear. We fear failing and we also fear succeeding. Our fear of failing often keeps us from fulfilling our goals; sometimes from even making that first attempt. But what about the fear of success?

Even though it may seem nutty, we often fear success as much, or even more than failure. We can let our fear of succeeding also keep us from our goals.

What could we possibly have to fear about becoming our slender selves you might wonder? Well, it is precisely that—becoming our slender selves—that might be the culprit. First there is the fear of the new, the different...the fear of change itself. Then, there is the fear of what does this change mean, how will it affect my life? Will people treat me differently? Will I be different? Will I get attention that I haven't had before? How will I deal with it? How will my friends and family react? Will they support me? Treat me differently?

Your fear of success may come in a different format...or you may not have any fear of success...or you might and not even be aware of it. Keep in mind these fears are on the subconscious level. It isn't that you would say "Yes!" if someone were to ask you "Are you afraid of losing weight?" In fact, you would more than likely say, quite emphatically, "NO!" But if you are making any kind of change in your life, it is common to wonder how it will affect the other people in your life and your relationship with them.

Case in point, I recently had a young man tell me that he "can't" focus on his health and fitness goals when he is around his friends because they do not share the same goals. So he continues to hang out with these friends and eat and drink with them. The rest of the time he follows his new path, but with these friends he is unwilling to change.

It may be he is afraid that his friends won't want to hang out with him if he orders water instead of beer...or has one beer instead of six...so he doesn't hang tough to his goals. Will his friends dump him if he doesn't partake in pizza feeding frenzies? I don't know...but I do know that he is afraid they will and he is, at this time, unwilling to risk that loss. This is how fear of success is manifesting for him.

Now, this fellow's goal is to have 6-pack abs. He is on a diet and following a strict workout regime to achieve those goals—except when he is around these friends. What he was expressing to me was regret at not being able to stick with his program. He was feeling guilty and bad about it. And because he is being so regimented about it, it is extremely obvious to his friends.

The good news is when you Refuse to Diet, you will go through this process naturally and you (and your friends) will have time to adjust to your new body. You won't be like I was when I did the liquid protein diet in college and lost 60 pounds over the summer and then felt like I was thrown to the wolves upon my return. You will have time to gain knowledge so you are able to deal with some of the emotional challenges that are triggered by our weight loss and our relationships with people.

Do keep in mind that you are changing, not just physically, but mentally too. If you want to change your body permanently then you will have to start with changing your mind. Like me, you may become more outgoing, more confident. You may actually begin to walk differently because you are no longer carrying around the excess baggage, both the physical and emotional. Your legs won't chafe, for one thing! You will have more energy and your new level of health and vitality will be apparent and attractive to others.

That doesn't mean that you are going to be approached for romance at every corner, but you will no longer be invisible. Instead of not being seen at all, or being looked at with pity, disgust or loathing, you may be viewed as "normal," or perhaps "attractive," or even "beautiful." This can be a very pleasant change; enjoy it and adjust to this new body—it can also be scary. Feel your emotions as you recognize your new shape, and how others react to it. If you do this you will have long-term success.

For many of us, food is soothing and our "friend." The subsequent fat is a way to protect us, to shield us. We may purposefully, albeit not fully consciously, get fat to create a protective barrier around ourselves. When that fat no longer serves to protect us, when we have gathered other support systems so we no longer need it, then we can let the fat go and it seems to literally start to melt away.

I know there are people out there who contend they are perfectly happy—they just like to eat. It is possible, certainly on the surface.

Just don't be surprised if there is more to it than that! That doesn't mean some hugely traumatic event happened in your life. Not everyone who is obese was molested as a child. But it is my understanding people don't tend to become addicted to drugs (including food) unless there is some sort of pain they are attempting to hide from or ignore.

I remember thinking that I was happy and okay. The truth was I had gotten so good at fooling others and myself that I believed the story. I forced myself to act like I was happy. I wanted to please others and they weren't happy when I was sad or angry, so I molded my face and my actions to suit their desires. I practiced my "happy face" and wore it so much that I had headaches most of the time.

Feeling Fat When it Just Isn't So

Whether you have reached your goal or still have a few, several or a lot of pounds to go, it can happen that we feel fat, frequently fatter than we actually are, even though we have already experienced some success in our weight loss journey. Why is that? How can I go from feeling fit and fabulous to fat and frustrated? Are there specific events that flip that switch? If yes, are they common to all of us involved in this struggle? Or are they our own fat "finger prints," unique and solely ours to bear?

Most people, women in particular, feel fat at some point in their lives. This may be based in fact or purely psychological. Sometimes it is in response to a normal healthy weight gain such as pregnancy, or it can be normal monthly hormonal fluctuations. Other times it may be from eating slightly too much at the holidays and having gained a pound or two.

What about those of us who have been making good, healthy choices and changes to our lifestyle, have dropped pounds and fat, are not pregnant (or haven't been pregnant) and can literally measure that our bodies are getting smaller...why do we sometimes still feel fat?

Having lost over 100 pounds I feel pretty fantastic most of the time. People definitely notice a difference in my appearance and energy level. My clothes were literally falling off my body so I've had to buy new. So why would I suddenly be on the brink of despair and feeling fat as ever? Obviously this was not a case of truth. I've spoken with experts in body image, psychology, nutrition, and brain chemistry and found that I am not alone in these feelings. The cause, the triggers, may vary from person to person, and certainly how we deal with the feelings has a tremendous impact on our overall health and continued success.

Semi-accurate Perceptions

We may have a temporary set-back. Perhaps our clothes feel a little tight, or the scale is up a bit, or maybe we have hit a plateau. So we feel fat, when it is possible we are just a bit bloated, or just having that temporary stall.

Best-selling author and public speaker, Brian Tracy talks about "Someday Isle"; I think this is a great image. We think that "someday I'll" do or be or feel in a certain way. For example, I will feel beautiful when I weigh 120 pounds, reach my goal weight, fit into those size 8 jeans. These may be great long-term goals, but they can set us up for feeling like failures, and fat, until we reach that specific goal. So, it may be accurate that you haven't reached that goal of being 120 pounds, and yet not accurate that you are fat. Or perhaps you are still "fat" as in you still want to lose 30 pounds (or 10 or 100), but that is placing the focus on what you have not yet accomplished instead of recognizing what you have done.

Inaccurate Perceptions

Taking the semi-accurate perception and distorting it further, we find people with a total disconnect between what their body feels like and looks like to them in the mirror, and how others perceive them. Case in point, after I did the liquid protein diet I was still fat in my mind. I kept seeing places where I could lose more fat. This was at the same time that I was in pain sitting because my bones had no padding. This is what the disorder anorexia is, a completely distorted picture of what you look like. Intellectually, I could tell something was strange when I needed a size 11-12 blouse to button around my neck and to cover my shoulders, but for a sleeveless tennis dress I only needed a size 4. Emotionally, I didn't recognize the distortion.

Inaccurate perceptions work both ways. We can also not see our growing lumps and thickening body when we gain weight. The problem is we don't see what our body really looks like. The severely anorexic and the fat person are just two manifestations of the same issue; two sides of the same coin. I know because I have been on both sides.

Unrealistic Expectations

Sometimes we just have unrealistic expectations of our body. There are two major paths here, the first is tied to the speed in which our results do, or do not, occur and the second is the physical result itself.

If we set a time frame goal for our weight loss result and we don't meet that goal, then we set ourselves up for disappointment, guilt and relapse. Setting realistic, flexible goals can help prevent this. Sometimes in our zeal in the beginning we'll set goals like "I'll lose 20 pounds in 2 months" which tends to be unrealistic for long-term healthy, sustained weight goals. Or we may set a more "reasonable" goal of dropping two pounds each week, not taking into account celebrations, vacations and plateaus.

Unrealistic expectations about physical results can be as simple as expecting to never experience challenges or plateaus. The other side of unrealistic expectations includes expecting to be a size that your body structure will not support. For example, I have strong, sturdy, (read large and muscular) legs. I will never have pinup girl or Miss America legs no matter how little I weigh. My bones are literally bigger around than some peoples' bones and muscles combined. Similarly, if you are blessed with an ample lower body, or pear shape, you will not morph into a lanky lean marathon body no matter what efforts you make.

Sure with diet and physical training we can modify our musculature and our size, but we do have genetic differences that we cannot entirely neutralize, which brings us to comparing ourselves to others.

Whether we are comparing our results in pounds lost, how quickly we lose weight, the method used to get results, or our actual bodies, comparing ourselves to others is rarely helpful. The reason it is not helpful is we tend to compare ourselves to someone "better" than us, someone who has had more success, someone who is "more beautiful." Instead of allowing someone else's successes to inspire and motivate us, we allow it to fuel our self-doubt and other negative emotions.

I am a stone sculptor, and so I am very aware there are all sorts of stones on this earth; one is not a better or more perfect stone than another. Some may be better suited for a particular function, or may be less common, and so society may place a higher value on it, but that is an artificial judgment created by comparisons. Truthfully, they are all beautiful in their own way. Some have been tumbled and polished in rivers or the ocean and so their colors are easily seen, while others need to sanded and polished to reveal their inner beauty. Some stones have a fine molecular structure and hold detail very well so are great for decorative carving. Other stones may be coarse but are very strong and are excellent for building. Others flake which can make them good cutting tools. All these stones have a purpose and a beauty. They are only "bad" when we try to force them into a purpose that is not suitable for their composition.

People are like that, too. One of the most wonderful things about human beings is our diversity. Some people have a more slender skeletal structure and therefore will be a different weight and size even though we may be the same height. I remember seeing Marie Osmond on the Oprah Winfrey show after she had lost some 50 pounds; she said she is a size 2/4 and that is a "healthy size" for her. I appreciated that she was admitting that there is a lot of pressure in her industry for her to be a size 0 (frankly, I don't understand how that can be possible, but that's a different subject) and that she has had to come to terms with the concept that she is larger than she "should" be according to that industry.

Marie and I are close to the same height, but that's about where the similarity ends. So while Marie was a size 14 at her heaviest, at almost fifty pounds overweight, a size 14 is a very healthy size for me. The point is we do not serve ourselves, or each other, by these comparisons. Go for what is healthy for you. Don't aspire to be a size 2/4 if your build demands a 10 or 12 or 16. Don't let anyone tell you there is some magic number on the scale or rack that you have to fit into.

Another interesting point about size and weight, Marie stated she weighs 125 pounds and is a size 2/4. My mother weighs 119 pounds and is a size 10. I don't know what size Oprah was at her "skinniest" but she will tell you in the photos where she is showing off her abs she was about 150 pounds. Keep all that in mind: the numbers are not the important thing. Use numbers to help gauge your own progress, but compare them only to your own numbers not someone else's.

As an artist I appreciate the differences in our shapes and sizes. When I worked as a lifeguard I found it fascinating how different and yet beautiful all the people were. You can't hide your differences at the pool under a bunch of clothes. Our roundness, the length of our limbs, the shape of our muscles all vary and are all beautiful, and they are all but superficial elements of what is our true beauty—that which is inside us!

Physical Reasons for Feeling Fat

Responses to a specific food item can also trigger a physical reaction that makes us feel fat. This is different from the over-full feeling we all experience after Thanksgiving. Here I'm referring to eating a normal serving size, or less, and still experiencing that overfull or bloated feeling.

When we were eating larger quantities of food and our clothes were tighter, we might not have noticed or felt the changes. Now that we are smaller the difference may be more noticeable. Clothes that were loose feel tight or we may feel sluggish as if we over indulged the night before. This could be our natural body rhythm and hormonal cycles, or it could signal a sensitivity or intolerance to a specific food. Not a true "allergy" in that you're not breaking out in hives or going into shock, but your body is just not processing this food item well. This could be a new development, or just a new awareness of an existing issue.

Common foods that cause these problems are dairy, wheat, gluten, refined sugar, salt, carbonation and alcohol. If you find you are experiencing bloat and/or sluggishness, ask yourself if you had any of these foods within the last day. Then try eliminating that food (or foods) as a test for a week and see if you start to feel better. Then try a little bit of that food after the elimination period and see how you feel. This elimination process can take time but identifying foods that really don't agree with you can pay off big down the road. You may still choose to have that food from time to time, but at least you won't be wondering why you don't feel so good, or why you feel fat when you do. Remember my friend with his reaction to ice cream? That's one example of having issues with food, and choosing to still indulge from time to time. He makes a conscious choice and is aware of the consequences of that choice.

Feeling Fat for Emotional Reasons

Emotions can also trigger feeling fat. This is not being a hypochondriac or having a psychosomatic issue, and it is not a matter of will power. Many of us have gained weight in the first place as a result of emotional triggers, from an overly critical parent, feeling alone and abandoned, to abuse—physical, verbal or sexual. Some people drink or take drugs as a coping mechanism to deal with these intense emotions. Other people get angry or even violent. And some of us eat. We are eating to push down the feelings because they are uncomfortable. Then we typically feel guilty, uncomfortable, or mad at ourselves, or just fat because we did eat. As a result we have built an association between the emotional cue and feeling fat.

I'm not a psychologist, but from my research I've learned it may still be too uncomfortable for us to feel the initial feeling, so we jump to the feeling that is easier for us to accept. For example, feeling abandoned may still hurt too much. Even though your rational adult mind may know that you weren't literally abandoned, that your parents were doing the best they could, maybe they both had to work to pay the bills, maybe one of your parents traveled a lot or was sick or even died. The intellect "knows" that your feelings are inaccurate and perhaps feels bad about it. The truth is, feelings are not subject to truth, they are perceptions.

Rather than admitting we feel like we were abandoned, we choose to eat comfort foods. And at first this worked...if it didn't we wouldn't have continued to eat in response to those feelings. Thus, we started a pattern of denying our feelings and eating instead. Later, we may not even be aware of the original feelings...we may think we have resolved the issue, or since we "know" the truth we may continue to discount the feeling.

So how do you know if you are feeling fat because of an emotional trigger? Take some time and write down what was going on for the day or two before your "fat feelings" came up. Did you talk to someone, have a visitor, see a movie, read a book. It could have even been an association that occurred on a shopping trip or hearing a song on the radio while driving in the car.

Emotional Eating

Even now, having gradually lost over 120 pounds I still feel the urge to eat when I am stressed, frustrated or sad. These are my most powerful triggers. For other people it could be fear, or even joy. What the emotion is really isn't important; the point is recognizing that there is a pattern of eating to hide or numb emotions rather than dealing with them.

Recognizing the pattern is the first step. The next step is to decide to be conscious of the pattern and to become a conscious eater. Recognition and awareness first and then develop other skills to handle the situations and emotions.

Refer to your own list of options from Chapter 5.

Awareness, Pattern Interrupt, Recognizing

The way to combat our "negative" thoughts which lead to over eating is with mega-doses of love. The first step to do that is to be aware of the negative thought and to break that habit. Tony Robbins calls it a pattern interrupt when you do something to help reinforce a change. I find it interesting that what we commonly call a light switch is actually called an "interrupter" because it interrupts the flow of electricity. You want to find your own "interrupter" to stop the flow of negative thoughts or comments that are flooding your mind.

A rubber band placed around your wrist is one idea for a simple interrupter you can use. Snap the band whenever you notice a negative thought to give yourself a small uncomfortable sensation or "negative association" and it will help remind you to not be negative.

Be sure to follow negative associations with a positive thought or affirmation and a gentle loving sensation called a "positive reinforcement". This could be as simple as rubbing the same wrist gently. In order for this to work you need to have at least one thing positive that you can say about yourself! I find it is best to have something ahead of time that you will say, rather than trying to think of something on the fly. So write a list of things that you are grateful that you do. If you absolutely cannot think of anything then you can use a general positive affirmation about your health such as "I am open to the possibility of attaining health." That is a wonderful attribute and believe it or not, there are many people who are not open to the possibility.

Practice your pattern interrupt, being sure to follow the negative association with positive reinforcement. In other words, don't just make yourself uncomfortable; give yourself a little non-food reward, too. Think about when you trained a puppy or a child. Did they learn best if you only scolded them? No, they did better and learned more quickly with a brief NO followed by positive direction delivered with love.

Avoid substitutes: don't eat anything for emotional reasons if you can avoid it...if you do, be aware that is what is going on. Don't substitute carrots for cookies. First of all, it really won't satisfy the urge...and while you have reduced calories you are still going through the motion, the habit, of eating instead of dealing with the issue. If you truly want to have permanent health you have got to start dealing!

No More Eating Mindlessly

You might be surprised to learn how much we eat that we aren't even aware of. There are hidden cues that determine how much and why people eat. These cues are mostly emotional and have little or no basis in our hunger or nutritional needs. Restaurants, supermarkets and other businesses spend a lot of money to learn what makes us eat more (and spend more money.) From packaging to color schemes, to music, it is all planned for their benefit, not our health.

It is up to us to be aware of what we are actually eating so that we are in control. Being aware of how much we really are consuming is a key facet to successfully losing weight—and keeping it off! In fact, by simply asking "Am I hungry?" or "Do I really want that?" before mindlessly grabbing that free sample or extra cookie, the average person can lose 10 - 20 pounds a year without making any other changes!

Other causes for eating mindlessly are emotional triggers caused by various stresses in our lives.

How many times have you had a rough day at the office and reached for a drink or treat as soon as you walked in the door? Or maybe you stopped on the way home and grabbed an ice cream.

You think you are hungry…but if you really stop and think about it your stomach isn't given you cues…you are eating because you are angry or tense or sad. Or maybe you are eating to celebrate.

The idea here is not to follow someone else's plan for you. This is about taking control back into your hands, empowering yourself, which includes making choices about what you eat, how much you move, and accepting the consequences for those choices.

There may be times when you consciously choose to overeat. Maybe it is a special occasion. If you go through the conscious thought process and you still choose to eat that cake, even the whole cake, then eat it and shut up about it. Don't whine, "I can't believe I did that!", or "Why did I do that?" just realize you chose to eat it and you will take the consequences—the sugar crash, possible weight gain, whatever. You may have had very valid reasons for eating what you did, and I for one am not going to judge you for it. My point is once you have done it, there is nothing to be gained by judging yourself for it either.

We have to start being more conscious about what goes into our mouth, but that doesn't mean we have to be perfect about it! What I have found is when we <u>consciously choose</u> to overeat, even if we are doing it to help numb our feelings, the mere fact that we have gone through the thought process enables us to eat less than we would if we were on auto-pilot.

In the beginning this will take a lot of effort to stop and think before every bite, before buying food and preparing it. By stopping yourself for even a split second you begin to engage your conscious mind and are starting to take control.

If you ask yourself "Am I physically hungry?" and the answer is no, then remember your plan, the list of other activities you can do rather than eating and try one or two of those. You may decide to come back and eat later, but you have broken the automatic reaction which is a fantastic victory!

Journaling

Many people find having a food journal is a big key to their weight loss success. I do find that it is a great tool to help keep my awareness "on"...to really be conscious about what I am eating. Especially as you are beginning on this journey and are looking at developing new skills.

In Chapter 5 we talked about journaling in terms of mindset: writing positive statements about yourself, and noting inspiring people you meet or read about. This can be the same journal, or if you prefer you can have a separate food journal. It really is up to you and what will help you the most. I like having things all in one place...I can see where I need some support, and I can also balance those places out by seeing my strengths and inspirations.

The food journal as covered in Chapter 7, was about establishing where you are...your benchmark. That is so important because we often really don't realize exactly where we are. Once you have established that benchmark you can use the food journal as a roadmap...it will help you see when you are on the path you want to be on, and where you tend to diverge.

As you progress on this journey you may find that you use your journal less frequently for recording what you eat...but if you find that you aren't losing weight and you think you should, it is an awesome tool to come back to. Think of it as a window into your world. The journal will help you to peer inside, to recognize what is going on in your head and heart.

As a refresher, the basics of a food journal are: it is a place to write down what you eat, and when you feel like eating—if you do eat, and if you don't eat; what are you feeling when you want to eat. It isn't so much a log of calories taken in...it is a tool to become aware of your emotional eating patterns.

The journal helps you to identify where your biggest challenges are, and gives you the opportunity to develop healthier habits to cope with your stress, anger, disappointment, boredom, and even your joy.

Ask yourself some very basic questions before each and every bite.

- Am I hungry?
- Is this food going to provide me with the nourishment my body needs?
- What am I trying to feed? (Is it my body, or is it my emotions?)
- How long has it been since I last ate?

If you aren't hungry, or you determine that food isn't going to be the right choice, then you have the perfect opportunity to break a habit. By consistently acting in a new way, you create a new habit that will result in weight loss.

Notes & Signs

Journals are great for delving into the <u>why</u> behind our eating patterns, but sometimes we need quick reminders that we are heading for unconscious eating. For this I use post-it notes and signs I put in various places to help remind myself to think before I eat.

For example, I have chocolate in the pantry and I have full permission to eat it...as long as I am making a conscious choice about it. So I have a note to myself on the shelf where the chocolate resides (I don't keep it at eye level, I keep it up high so I have to actually seek it out.) On the note I ask myself if this is what I really want. What do I really want to feed at the moment? I'm amazed at how frequently just seeing that little note gives me pause enough that I think about it and decide, "You know what? I don't really want any chocolate." Other times I will note that I really just want the creamy texture melting in my mouth and by reading that note it reminds me to savor it and make the most of the experience.

Other great places for notes and reminders are on the fridge, the computer monitor, in with my lunch, on the door so I see it when I walk out, and on the bathroom mirror. Find places where you can use some inspiration, encouragement, or just a reminder to stop and think before eating and put your notes there. Remember to keep the notes loving and thoughtful. These notes are not intended to be a harsh "Stop or you will die" message; it is about becoming aware and loving your body to health.

Choosing Foods

"Success, Failure: Choose"

~Brent Payne

The second step in taking back your life is choosing foods. I believe most of us know what to eat and what not to, so I'm not going to go deep into nutrition. If you need some guidance in this area there are lots of nutrition experts out there; my personal recommendation is my friend Dr. Linda—she knows more about nutrition and how the body processes foods than just about anybody. I mentioned in Chapter 6 how Dr. Linda helped my mother review her blood tests...well, she also guided my mom through the minefield of being diagnosed diabetic...what that really means, and eased a lot of her fears about it, while empowering her to take control of her health. You can find how to contact Dr. Larson for a consultation in the Resources section in the back of this book.

I talk about food as my drug of choice throughout this book. More specifically, my drug of choice was ice cream, the more chocolaty and creamy the better. But I was not an exclusive overeater. If I ate pizza, I ate half the "family" size. I even overate when it came to vegetables and meat. I ate pretty much like it was Thanksgiving every day, so portion control was a big issue for me.

But what really got me into trouble wasn't my meals, it was the unconscious eating. You can use this exercise at any point and I encourage you to use it over and over again throughout the day. If you do that, I guarantee you will shed fat and improve your health. Regular repetition of this new behavior will ultimately lead it to become your new automatic response replacing your old, self-destructive patterns.

Success Tool

This exercise is very simple, it is a question, "Is this choice leading me towards my goal (success) or not (failure)?"

Most of the time, you will choose success over failure. Sometimes you will consciously say, "No, this choice is not moving me towards my goal and I am <u>still</u> choosing to divert from my goal by doing this." It is all about making a conscious choice.

So how do I use this tool in my day-to-day life? In the morning I start with the basic intention of choosing success today. Don't presume it—claim it! "I choose success today! I make choices today that move me closer to my health goals."

> "I didn't gain this weight in one weekend. It was one more bite that did me in."
>
> ~Zig Ziglar

Sometimes we have to make the same choices repeatedly, which makes sense—after all we made the same unhealthy choices over and over to get to be fat, didn't we? It is about being conscious about how we feel and making conscious decisions that support our goals.

I incorporate these into my notes so I see them and remind myself to claim my success on a daily basis. Success/Failure: Choose. Short, easy to grasp, and filled with meaning.

How to Apply Success/Failure: Choose in Your Life

If you tend to skip breakfast, ask if that is going to move you closer to your goals. It won't for me. With decades of dieting under my belt I have trained my body to not register "hungry" very often, but I know that I perform better—and eat less—if I have breakfast, including protein, in the morning. I'm not a slave to the notion that I have to <u>start</u> my day with breakfast, it may be that I have my breakfast an hour or two or even three later, but I will generally have a meal early in the day because I know it serves me to. Not because I "should", because I <u>feel better</u> when I do.

How about exercising, how often do you feel like skipping out on that routine? When I don't feel like moving I repeat the question, or just think Success/Failure: Choose. Often that is enough to get me moving.

Someone brings doughnuts to the office, Success/Failure: Choose. Lunch time, do I eat the healthy food I brought, go out to eat with my co-workers, run to the drive through, or skip lunch and work? Success/Failure: Choose. It's the bosses' birthday and so cake appears, Success/Failure: Choose. The candy jar on your co-workers desk has just been refilled, Success/Failure: Choose.

Is This Just About Willpower?

To some people this may seem like trying to evoke willpower, but it is much different from that. The motivation behind it is different, and the level of control is different. Willpower implies for me that I am actually weak and have to struggle against something that is bigger than I am. Success/Failure: Choose reminds me that I have the choice in everything I do which is extremely empowering. But if the words bother you, then change them!

It isn't about never having a slice of cake—in fact you may decide that having a piece of cake is part of moving you towards your health goals. I find it very important to be able to celebrate with friends, family and co-workers, and food is a part of celebrations. My goal is to have a "normal" relationship with food, so sometimes the right choice for me is to have that treat. When I do, I also realize that if my goal is to have a "normal" relationship with food, then I deserve to savor every morsel and know that I can have it whenever I want, so there is no need to wolf it down or have three and four servings.

> "Preserving health by too strict a regimen is a wearisome malady."
>
> ~François duc de La Rochefoucauld, ©1650

The word "failure" can be a stumbling block, but it is not to indicate that YOU are a failure if you choose to divert temporarily from your goal. It is really just a reminder that by making that choice I will be delaying my arrival. As long as most of the time I choose success, I will achieve my goal, and if it takes me a bit longer that is okay, I'll get there!

This is not about deprivation, that's what will power is about. I love food. I love to travel and I love trying new foods and flavors when I travel. So my health goal includes celebrations and food exploration. When I am in Paris I will have pastries with my coffee, I wouldn't feel healthy and normal if I said I couldn't enjoy any pastries in France!

Because I am enjoying the food, I actually have found that there are times when I don't eat it all. I've gotten pretty good at splitting entrees and desserts. Most restaurants in the US serve portions fit for a lumberjack even when there is not a tree in sight. If I can't split it, either because I'm alone or my meal partner wants something different I usually take half home.

Tip: if the portion comes and it is large, cut it in half first!

What if I forget the Success/Failure: Choose question?

Don't sweat it if you forget to ask the question from time to time, but if you find you are forgetting frequently then write yourself some notes. Abbreviate it as S/F:C if you want—most people will think it refers to some computer program that you are working on! I have my screen saver set to "I Choose Success" and no one else has to know what I mean by that.

Chapter 9: Food Challenges

"God gives every bird its food, but He does not throw it into its nest."

~J.G. Holland

Okay, since you can't eliminate food and expect to live, we know we will have to face some challenges around what goes in our mouths. Some of the common challenges we face are cravings, compulsions, good nutrition, and special events.

Cravings

Cravings are one of the number one challenges and one that we feel we have no control over! People ask me all the time, "How did you get over the sugar cravings?" or "How do I stop the urge to eat carbohydrates?"

> "Feed me now, or I'll kill you!"
>
> ~Dr. Mehmet Oz, identifying one of the three basic categories of sugar cravings.

Cravings can be a sign of an addiction. Our body is signaling us that it wants something that it thinks it needs, even when we know intellectually that this thing is bad for us. No one believes that meth is good for your body but once you become addicted to it, the addiction is stronger than you are, or at least for most people.

The "feed me now" craving is typically a response to low blood sugar.

Sugar can also be an addiction, fortunately not one with as dire consequences as meth, but it can be a deadly addiction just the same, over time. For many people, cravings are the single biggest stumbling block to weight loss success. Whether is it is refined sugars found in cakes and sweets, or the simple carbohydrates found in breads and pastas which are immediately converted to sugars in the body, sugars are the main culprit. Sugar gives us a burst of energy which is then followed by a drop or crash when our blood sugar level drops back down. To combat that drop we eat more sugar or drink a soda, anything to give us that artificial energy boost. Just like the meth addict, we are constantly seeking our next high, only ours is easier to score!

When you are feeling cravings you can first look to see if there is an emotional reason behind the craving. When they come on really suddenly that is generally the case. More of a slow onset can be purely physical, like you had a lot of simple carbs and now the floor just dropped out from under you. And you can also have hormonal issues that set up cravings, especially in women around their menstrual cycle or during pregnancy.

Dr. Oz suggests you suck on a Tic Tac to stop major cravings, but that doesn't do anything for me. His next suggestion is one that I completely agree with, and is supported by Dr. Nicholas Perricone in the *Perricone Prescription*, and that is to eat more frequently. My ex-husband use to claim he got PMS three times a day: pre-meal syndrome. If you find that you get grumpy, irritable, or fatigued between meals then try the mini meal approach rather than reaching for the caffeine or sugar to temporarily boost you back up.

One of the keys to dealing with the physical cause of cravings is to eat on a regular basis. A lot of people think they should restrict themselves to eating only once or twice a day. Studies show that you will actually consume more calories if you eat this way. You are better off have four to six mini-meals every day, eating every few hours. This keeps your blood sugar more stable and will help keep the cravings at bay.

When we allow ourselves to eat excessive sugar, especially the pure stuff like white sugar and high fructose corn syrup, we are setting ourselves up for a crazy ride. This ride is not fun for us, and is no picnic for our friends, family, and co-workers either. After the sugar high there is an inevitable blood sugar crash. Rather than "solving" the crash problem by rushing to get more sugar, we can get natural sugars in the form of fruits and vegetables which break down more slowly in our blood stream. This will give us a slower, more consistent blood sugar level.

By choosing fruits and vegetables, we can have the sweet tastes without Mr. Toad's Wild Ride. I'm personally convinced that a large number of people who are on anti-depressants really need to be off sugar—or at least greatly reduce the amount they consume. I can say that because I was one of them. When you are depressed you grab anything that helps boost you up, and sugar will artificially do that— for a while.

So, especially if you are on anti-depressants, I suggest you reduce your sugar intake. I'm not saying you have to eliminate it entirely; one of my key concepts is that no foods are forbidden. Just try curbing your sugar intake for a while and see how you feel. I still love sweets, but I don't love how I feel when I eat too much of them. I have been able to break the cycle of sugar addiction, so I know it is possible. I can now have treats without going off the deep end into a binge.

We all have urges, to eat things that are bad for us, to smoke, or to gamble, but most people have a level of control over those urges. For those of us who do not, these urges can become compulsions that seem to have control over us. We don't feel we have the power to stop ourselves, or we may not even remember participating in the compulsive act.

Simply by learning the reason behind the compulsion, or even "just" cravings, can help free us from it. It *may* always be there to a certain degree, but we can probably learn to live with it. And with practice and changing our mindset, I believe we can completely liberate ourselves from feeling controlled by these compulsions.

Eat Often

Don't skip meals. Dieters skip meals in a misguided attempt to reduce the number of calories they take in every day. This has been proven to backfire and actually people who skip meals tend to consume more calories on a daily basis. We discussed the challenge of carbohydrate cravings earlier, and one of the biggest tools you can use to help fight carb cravings is to eat smaller meals, with protein of some kind, four to six times every day.

Diet Is a Four Letter Word

You don't have to go on a diet...in fact my entire premise is you don't want to go on a "diet" because diets don't work. We've already covered that. I've also discussed how your mind is the primary weight loss mechanism. Keeping that in mind, pun fully intended, let's talk about food as a weight loss tool...including diets and diet foods (no, say it isn't so!)

Nutrition: sometimes we need to educate ourselves in order to ensure we are getting adequate nutrition. We are changing our eating habits and learning to listen to our bodies. Years of ignoring the body's cues can make it difficult to interpret what it is trying to tell us it needs. By knowing some good nutritional basics, and then paying attention to how you feel physically, mentally, and emotionally after you eat will greatly assist you in learning this new "language."

Sometimes food tools can help us temporarily while we are learning new habits. Other times we like them for their convenience and we may use them frequently. No matter what, it is important to remember they are just a tool, not the answer. They are not a "magic bullet." The magic is in you and your mind.

No Forbidden Foods

While you are becoming a more conscious eater, and changing your mindset and habits, you may not want to stock up on foods that have tended to send you on a binge in the past. I call these "trigger foods." It is very likely that later you will be able to have them around and not feel their toxic pull, but when you are first changing your mindset the old habits may be stronger than the new desire. I see no reason to "test" yourself. Keep in mind **you can have anything you truly desire.** The key is to be conscious about what you are eating, and to know that it is what you truly desire.

So, if you truly want that bread, or chocolate, or chips, or in my case, ice cream, then go out and get yourself some. I found that by giving myself permission to have it and yet having it be a conscious effort to go out and get it, that gave me the time and space to make a conscious decision about eating—rather than having it be a knee jerk reaction. Frequently that was all I needed to decide that I really didn't want it after all.

If you do go to buy some food or drink item, then take the time and really enjoy it! Make it an event. Don't stuff it down. That is the big clue right there. If you find that you race to the store and want to slam the food down as fast as possible, then you are definitely eating for emotional reasons, not because of any real physical need.

Fast Food

If time is one of your biggest challenges (and who doesn't have this challenge) you will want to have an arsenal of healthy foods you can get quickly. Ideally we should take time to eat and enjoy every bite. We all "know" this, we also know that realistically we just don't live this way, and that is probably not going to change. Have leisurely eating as a goal as often as possible, and also have some lifelines in place for the times when you just don't have even 5 minutes.

If you go to a fast food restaurant, check out their menus. Go sometime when you aren't hungry. Just make it a research trip; another tool in your weight loss success toolbox. Most fast food restaurants have some grilled options. Salads are generally also available, but two things about their salads: if they come with dressing on them they are going to be heavy in fat and calories without your control. This isn't about not being able to have dressing...it is about tasting the food and controlling quantities, so if you can't control the amount of dressing on the salad then it may not be your best fast food choice.

Keep Things On Hand

Even though you are going to be getting the food quickly and probably eating it fast too, be aware of what you are eating. Give yourself a minute to be fully conscious of your choices, including the tastes and textures. If you just gulp them down you will not feel satisfied and you will tend to over eat. Have portions predetermined when you figure out these foods. That way you don't go overboard when you grab and run. That is especially easy to do when we slip into unconscious eating mode.

Some of My Favorite Quick Foods

Nuts: for best health choose raw over roasted. I like a variety of nuts, sometimes one type "straight up" and at other times a blend. So I buy bags of raw nuts and mix as desired or not. Nuts contain "good fats" and are nutritionally very dense so you don't need a lot. I love almonds, pecans, hazelnuts and Brazil nuts. Pine Nuts are also personal favorites. I keep a jar in the cupboard with a mixture of various nuts and some raisins (I select the 100% fruit, no sugar.) This lets me grab a small snack that has protein and some sweetness, and it is also something I can carry with me if I'm going to be away from the house.

Portion Control Tip: it doesn't take very many nuts to count as a serving, so it can be really easy to eat three to four servings at a whack. Two easy portion control tools I use are the small "Dixie" cups or soy sauce dishes. I prefer the dishes for around the house; I like that they feel like little plates and they are more fun. I psychologically feel more satisfied when I eat from them then the cups, but the cups are easier to transport.

String Cheese: I love this! I enjoy peeling little threads off the string and savoring the pieces. Portion control is easy here since they come prepackaged. I have one and then if I am still hungry later I can have another.

Red Peppers: I know this sounds funny, but these are one of my favorite foods—seriously! I love the sweetness and the crunch. I also love that I can cut them up and keep the strips in a container so they are quick to get at.

Prewashed Salad: this is a huge boon for me in food prep time savings, and makes having a salad a possibility when I might otherwise not have the time to make one.

Hard Boiled Eggs: a good, lean protein with built in portion control. They are great for eating as is, or in a salad.

Artichoke Hearts: I buy both the plain and the marinated kinds and mix them together. Then I allow a little of the oil to drip on my salad and use that as my dressing. I love the flavor, but just the marinated ones are too much. I started off mixing them 50-50, but as my tastes have changed I really like less oil, so now I use mostly (or 100%) the plain variety. Then I can also add my own oil and vinegar because it gives me the most control.

Premade Foods: a general comment about premade foods, including shakes and bars, you are going to have to read the labels and really pay attention to your own body on these!

Protein Shakes: I like a protein shake for breakfast. I enjoy the light, yet nourished, feeling I get from a shake, as opposed to a big breakfast. However, I have found it is critical to be very careful when selecting a shake; I have not found one that is premixed (meaning a can of liquid) that works for me. Most shakes have a lot of sugars in them and I have actually found that they will spike my blood sugar, which is a really bad way to start my day. I enjoy the rich taste and having some "chocolate" but the sugary ones set me up on a roller coaster just like I was eating a donut! Other shakes I've found have caffeine or other ingredients that give me the jitters—so, again, read the labels and pay attention to your own body.

When you look for shakes and bars, look for ones with a balance of protein, carbs and fats. Roughly 2 carbs to 1 protein is a good balance. This helps keep your blood sugar balanced, so you don't have that spike and the subsequent crash. For women, fats should be about ½ the grams of the protein.

Shakes that I've tried with success: Venus Wellness Formula, sold by Isagenix and My Victory, sold by Pharmanex. The Venus Wellness Formula is for women; Isagenix also has a Mars Wellness Formula for men. Both the Isagenix lines are specially formulated by Dr. John Gray and are different from the regular Isagenix line.

Dr. Linda has reviewed both these products and they have her 'seal of approval.' I personally prefer the Venus Formula and this is also the product that Dr. Linda personally uses.

The Wellness Formula shakes are not "diet foods"...Dr. Gray designed them to balance brain chemistry and they serve as a meal replacement. According to John, when our brain chemistry is balanced we will naturally shift to our best weight; if your body should carry less fat you will drop fat; if you need to gain weight you will do that. I had a hard time initially grasping this concept. Based on my past education and experience I thought there had to be two different shakes to achieve these goals. That was because I was coming from a "diet" perspective: if you want to drop weight you drink a low-cal shake, if you want to gain muscle you drink a high-cal shake. That is what makes these shakes so unique...and, again, not a "diet" product!

I was enjoying having shakes every morning for breakfast, and I was dropping weight (and fat.) I began to wonder if perhaps my mindset theory about weight loss was wrong, or flawed. Maybe the shakes were the "magic bullet" that people were looking for. That was exciting and scary at the same time. I became a little afraid that if the shake was the real reason I was losing weight, then if I stopped drinking them I would either stop losing weight or even gain the weight back.

I didn't like that idea at all! First of all, it went against my idea of not dieting. After all, if I am only able to lose weight because I'm drinking this shake (or eating "that bar"...) then I become dependent upon that product and I don't have control over it. What if I want to go on a long trip...would I have to carry the shake with me? Will I have to drink the shake the rest of my life? What if I decide I want a break? What if the company changes the formula, or goes out of business?

I decided to run a personal experiment and go off the products. I still drank lemon and water in the morning...I bought fresh lemons and squeezed them. I still did my 15 minute exercise routines. I still did my affirmations, my journaling. But I had no shakes at all. I did this for six months. I still lost weight.

Hurray! I felt very validated...and totally in control. Now I could go back to drinking the shakes as I desired, knowing they are not the cause of my weight loss. I drink them because I like the ease, the convenience, the taste, the light feeling I have...and because it is a meal I really don't have to think about. That works great for me!

I also know that I can go on vacations and enjoy whatever foods I encounter. I don't have to tote canisters of products in my suitcase. What is convenient at home is not necessarily convenient while on the road.

These days I eat pretty much like a "normal" healthy person (whatever "normal" means!) and I happen to most days choose to enjoy a very healthy meal replacement shake for my breakfast.

Do I recommend these shakes? Totally. Because they are quick and easy...and you have one less meal to think about they are fantastic. They are nutritious and taste great. I do not feel that way about all shakes.

I looked at lots of different shakes. The ones that I found that had a similar balance and provide the nutrition and brain chemistry benefit are the Venus Wellness Formula (Mars Wellness Formula for men) and My Victory. The Wellness Formula products, because they have a different formulation for men and women are my first choice, but a good second choice is My Victory. The only downside to the VWF is it only comes in chocolate...not really a downside for most chocoholics, but if you want a vanilla base then try My Victory.

I've included some "recipes" in the Resources section that you can try with any shake powder...just remember to read the labels to make sure you are getting a good balance of protein/carbs/fat...that's why I like the Wellness Formula and My Victory shakes...I know I'm getting a healthy balance that I need to be my best.

Note: neither the Wellness Formula products nor My Victory are available in stores. Refer to the Resources section in the back to learn how you can order them.

Bars: be especially careful with bars, even those billed as protein bars or meal replacement bars. Many of them have little more nutritional value than a candy bar. Again, read the labels. If you find one that has a good protein level and low sugars (remember the 2 carbs to 1 protein ratio) and has a taste you enjoy, than have a couple on hand. The danger I found with bars is it is super easy to grab them and eat them like a candy bar—which isn't changing your habit or mindset.

Foods to be Extra Aware of

Okay, this is not a "diet" book, but it is about gaining health, so I would be remiss if I didn't mention a few foods that it would be better if we reduce our intake of. Notice I say reduce rather than eliminate. As I have said before, I don't believe in "forbidden foods" for psychological reasons—by making something off-limits the kid in us will rebel and want it more, which can result in binges, and ultimately weight gain, rather than weight loss success.

I watch out for the following because they are really empty calories: white flour, sugar, high-fructose corn syrup...pretty much anything labeled "syrup." Also on my list to avoid are artificial sweeteners, especially aspartame...which is in a lot of diet foods. I happen to be allergic to it and it gives me major headaches. I have spoken to lots of other people who never put it together and are surprised how their headaches go away once they stop taking aspartame. There are also several studies that indicate that eating artificial sweeteners stimulates the taste buds for sweets and we actually want to consume more, not less! So if you are craving sweets, cut out the fake stuff! Most people are better off having some real sugar, but if you have specific health concerns (like diabetes) talk to your doctor, or schedule a consult with Dr. Linda to see what is best for you.

Holidays, Vacations, Special Events and Celebrations

Holidays and family gatherings are huge challenges for most of us. Have you ever geared up for the anticipated overeating by cutting back before hand, only to find that not only did you pig out over the event, the pig out fest went on long after it was over? Then did you go into punishment mode, "I'm so stupid," "I can't believe I ate all that crap"?

Again, my philosophy is there are no forbidden foods. Realize that you can enjoy sampling all the foods you want, and if you choose to enjoy something, relax about it and enjoy it without guilt or punishment. Holding onto the guilt only allows you to hold onto the fat, too. Enjoy life, including food. When you are not enjoying the food, when you no longer tasting it, then stop eating it.

Naturally thin people do this and you can too, by giving yourself permission to eat anything you want.

I saw a movie over the holidays about a food critic who went from restaurant to restaurant, ordering many meals a day. She survived this without gaining weight by only have a bite or two of everything, enough to get the flavors. A bite or two might not sound like much, but remember she was eating at many, many different restaurants every day...and she ate a bit or two of everything, including the carbs and desserts.

I mention this movie because I found it to be very inspiring. It really goes to show (even though it was a movie) that you can eat whatever you want. The idea is to savor food and get the flavors. Many people will say you just can't lose weight if you eat out a lot or travel for business. It just isn't true. Remember that you are in control. You can choose foods that will keep your blood sugar in balance. You can choose smaller portions. If you are somewhere that you can take part of the meal home—great, do that. If you aren't then don't let the adage of not letting food "go to waste" put it on YOUR waist! Eat what you want. Enjoy it. And then stop.

I have found that I can, and do, eat whatever I want. Yes, I want less volume and I want fewer sweets, but I still love chocolate and will often save room for dessert by taking some of my meal home (or sharing it with a friend) so that I can also enjoy the finale.

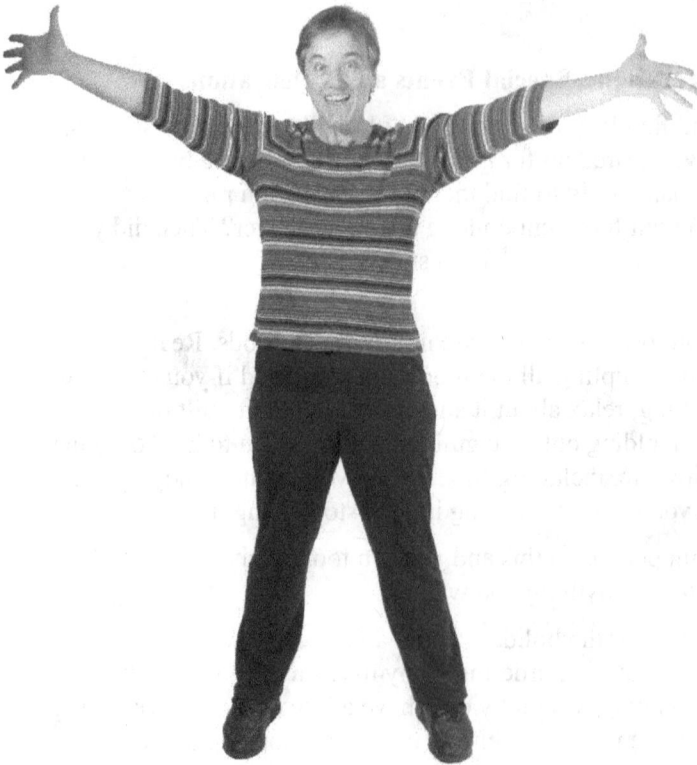

Chapter 10: People: Challenges and Helpers

"God grant me the serenity to accept
the people I cannot change, the
courage to change the one I can, and
the wisdom to know it's me."

~Author Unknown

When People Are a Challenge

To some people, you may even seem like a different person...which in a very real sense you are in the process of becoming.

They Treat You Differently

Remember when I lost a lot of weight in college and suddenly I got a lot of attention from guys? Well, to be honest...it kind of pissed me off. Guys who didn't even seem to see me before, were suddenly talking to me and asking me out. I remember being angry and thinking "I'm the same person on the inside, where were you last year?" While that was true in part, in another way it was not true. I was actually more confident and outgoing. I felt better and had more energy. My body radiated a different aura because I was taking better care of it.

Realize that you <u>are</u> changing. You cannot be the same exact person and successfully lose weight. Yes, some people will respond to you differently, and you may have to learn some new skills to handle it.

No Acknowledgment of Your Success

There will also be people who do not treat you differently, who do not acknowledge or appreciate the changes you make. Most of these people will not be a problem. Some of these people are unconscious, and others are not sure what to say. Perhaps they just saw your inner self all along and the outer shell just isn't that important to them. Those are some pretty cool people to have around! If you really want them to acknowledge your results, you will probably have to tell them!

Saboteurs

You may experience people in your life who on the surface seem to be happy for you, who say they are proud of your results, but who sabotage your efforts. Know these are people who probably don't like change, or they are simply jealous, or afraid. It may be that you are growing independent of them, and they fear they will lose you, or they may not like the attention you are getting. Maybe your spouse or boyfriend feels some jealousy, or maybe a girlfriend used to get the attention that you are now getting, or they may just not like that you are succeeding because they are internalizing it as an indictment of their own failures. It could also be because you are no longer numbing yourself with food and you are actually owning what is going on in your life, you may be feeling and expressing your emotions more, which may make them uncomfortable.

If you have a saboteur in your midst, you deserve to cut them off at the pass. If it is a close friend or family member you may want to have a real heart to heart conversation with them and see if you can resolve the issue. For some people, there will be "friendships" that do not survive. Realize that if they can't handle that you are getting healthy, then they are not a true friend, and you have to put your health first over their comfort.

Friends and Family May Face Fears, Too

Even if they do not actively sabotage your efforts, your friends and family may experience fears that center around your weight loss. As much as they love you, and want you to be happy and to succeed, your relationship to those around you will adjust when you lose weight.

What was your role in the relationship in the past? Were you the "happy fat girl"? Well, if you are no longer the "fat girl" who are you? How do you fit in? If you were one of a crowd of fat people, they may want to pull you back to the "good old days" when you ate and drank to excess together. They may wonder if your life no longer revolves around that, if you will still be friends. Of course you can still be friends with some of them. And the people who truly love you will be there. However, realize that friendship is a two-way street that you don't have complete control over. If you have enough things in common besides excessive eating and drinking, then it is likely you will remain friends even though this friendship will no doubt evolve.

Whether they begin to see you differently, or feel threatened by the changes in your appearance, when you lose weight gradually not only do you get to adjust to your new body, but so do your loved ones.

Letting People Go

Not all of our friends are friends for life. Sometimes it is time to let people pass out of our lives, and you deserve to give yourself permission about that. Even if they are not actively sabotaging your health efforts, if the only connection you have with people is about food and eating, then you may have to move on.

This is easier to admit and see how critically important it is when you are talking about drug addicts or alcoholics, but really it is the same. In some ways it is harder if food has been your drug of choice because it is legal and so readily available. Be strong for yourself.

Friends and Supporters

People may be some of our biggest challenges, but they can also be some of our biggest assets in our journey to health!

You are surrounding yourself with affirmations, positive books and changing your behaviors, but don't forget your friends, family and supporters can be some of your biggest success tools. Don't be afraid to ask for help. Tell people how they can help you, don't make them guess.

One of the tenets of Twelve Step programs like Alcoholics Anonymous and Overeaters Anonymous is letting go and asking for help from a higher power. When you ask for help, you may want to include whatever higher power you choose: it might be your internal wisdom, the universe, God, angels, or a departed loved one. Get help wherever it works for you.

There are people who inspire us because of their own weight loss or their health challenges and how they are moving forward. The very real nature of Ruby Gettinger, who has a reality show on the Style Channel, serves as an inspiration to many people. I love that she is so open and human! I really admire that she was out there living her life, even before she started to lose weight.

That is an important concept that a lot of people ignore. Don't put off living your life until you reach a certain weight or size. Live your life now. Be the person you want to be, the person that you are deep inside. Then you will start to match that person on the outside.

Coaches

You may decide you want some additional help or education either in terms of exercise or nutrition. There is nothing wrong with that at all.

A lot of us know the basics about what to eat...it is just that we don't necessarily apply what we know! However, if you don't, then get some good nutritional information. Find someone who can help guide you in a way that fits your life. In other words, don't work with a gourmet vegan if you are currently a fast food queen! You might get there someday, but for now that is probably too big a leap.

Yes, be open to new ideas, but if you have 15 minutes to prepare meals on average, don't work with someone who will expect you to spend an hour. It won't be a good fit, will frustrate you both, and you won't keep it up. Let yourself evolve over time...this isn't a sprint—it is for life!

Work Out Buddies

Work out buddies can be awesome when you choose people who encourage you and who have the same types of goals you do.

I suggest having a couple of different buddies. If you are walking as a major part of your movement program then have a walking partner who is at a similar pace, or choose a path that allows you to see each other periodically for support even if you can't match stride for stride.

Social aspects to your routine are great, they can really add to the fun, but don't let the talking be the priority.

One of the best things about having a workout buddy is the camaraderie. Share laughter and smiles and breathe in some good clean fresh air.

Support Groups

Many people really benefit from having a support community—a group of like-minded individuals who understand the journey that you are on. Some people have a group like that, either in their existing friends and family members, or they can join a local group, maybe Weight Watchers or Overeaters Anonymous. For others, they don't have the support available or they don't have time to attend meetings...or they don't like the structure. For them, online communities are great.

This is one of my goals with http://www.RefuseToDiet.com, to create an online community to help connect people to achieve weight loss and health goals without a strict "this is the one and only diet that will work" approach. I see this as a place where we can all share our experiences, our successes, and motivate and support one another. I hope that you will join us!

Chapter 11: Setbacks and Other Challenges

"Let us rise up and be thankful, for if
we didn't learn a lot today, at least we
learned a little, and if we didn't learn
a little, at least we didn't get sick, and
if we got sick, at least we didn't die;
so, let us all be thankful."

~Buddha

Setbacks

The path to our ideal weight and health is not a straight line. There will be setbacks along the way. For me when I started it was easy in the beginning. I lost twenty pounds right away and I was proud of my accomplishments. Then I got derailed. I went to a conference and one of the speakers was a health and fitness guru. He challenged everyone to participate in his program for 12 weeks and transform our bodies. The program sounded great and the energy in the room was high as we all vowed to accept his challenge. Ironically, that was my downfall.

Suddenly I was no longer doing this for me and I was no longer focused on my mind. I was back in diet mode, setting goals, and doing it for someone else, the group or the guru, it didn't really matter, it wasn't for me.

Whether it was that diet or any diet, it was wrong for me and I stopped losing weight. I struggled for months with it. I did lose some weight, but it was so hard...I felt deprived...I struggled with cravings...and I gained the weight back.

Then another setback, my father died. I ate through my grief. My belief in my ability to choose health had vanished.

Ultimately, my father's death was a big catalyst for change. After several months of "griezing," grief laden grazing, I finally asked myself, "How long are you going to use your father's death as another excuse to not lose weight?" It could have been a slightly different question a few years earlier, but it was always about making an excuse. And I had lots of them, losing jobs, break ups, divorce, more job loss, death of pets, moving, new jobs, fear, stress, loneliness.

Shortly after I turned 48 I asked myself that question and I decided the answer was "no longer."

"Coincidentally" (I don't really believe in coincidences), my partner Cathy and our friend Dr. Linda attended a conference less than two weeks after my birthday. This conference was where they first met Dr. John Gray and learned about his wellness program.

I will confess that my first response to their enthusiasm was complete and utter skepticism. When they said he had a shake that was aimed for balancing brain chemistry which had the added side benefit for some people of losing weight, all I heard was "shake" and I said I'd "been there, done that." Then when they told me they had arranged for me to visit John at his ranch...well...I was furious, I was hurt...I felt like I was being sent to a fat farm! I took their love-filled intentions as criticism, as an attack, an indication that I wasn't good enough as I was.

Self-doubt

These reactions to their loving intentions were because I doubted my ability to lose weight, and because I didn't believe I was worthy of achieving health. Even though I had said I was not going to let more excuses get in my way, I still wasn't completely convinced I could do it.

Self-doubt is something that affects so many of us. We don't feel good enough, smart enough, talented enough, you-fill in-the-blank-enough. This underlying current keeps us from enjoying our experiences. We have a constant need for approval from someone outside of ourselves. This is a huge challenge that affects our body-image and weight loss. I don't know where this need comes from, but I know it is very common among women of my generation.

This self-doubt also applied to writing this book, "Who am I to write this book?" and then I realized that I am the only one who can write this book, because it is my story. I don't need a fancy diploma on the wall to give me permission to write my story. I have the education of personal experience. Who is better suited to write about successful weight loss; someone who studied it in others, but has never known what it is like to struggle, be overweight, fail and succeed, or the person who has gone through the pain and come through it stronger? Each person has a valid perspective, but if merely studying what others did brought successful health, then there would be little need for this book.

> "There is a dance that occurs between being and doing, but for most of my life I let Doing be in control."
>
> ~Laurie Tossy

This book is less about what to DO and more about how to BE. There is a dance that occurs between being and doing, but for most of my life I let Doing be in control. It was by relaxing and letting Be lead that I finally was able to do the things that led to having my healthy body.

What does it mean to allow "Be" to lead? It means getting my spirit in alignment first. I call it mind, but it is more than that—and certainly not my brain. This is not an intellectual pursuit. I knew for years what to eat, what not to eat, how much exercise to do, etc. in order to be healthy. I would even go through periods where I actually did those things, but until my being-ness was in alignment with that of a healthy, happy, slender person, I couldn't keep it up. That is why diets fail. They focus on tasks, on Doing. A diet can only succeed if it is built on a foundation of Being.

Once you have that foundation, there are lots of diet and exercise programs that can assist in educating you, if that is something you want. Perhaps they can speed up the process, but the diet is secondary to your being, your mindset, your attitude, your beliefs. This is the real work, changing your thoughts and beliefs. When you do that, your actions will naturally follow. Be leads. Do follows. The result is a beautiful dance of health.

Trusting Self

We all have an inner wisdom that if we trust it, will guide us to our ideal health. Most of us have distrusted and ignored these messages for so long that we either don't hear them or don't believe them.

So while we have this guidance, it may be overpowered by other messages. Overpowered by either a cacophony of conflicting calls, or practically silent, true messages may be drown out by the stronger, false messages that we have nurtured over the years.

Why the stronger messages don't just disappear with a decision:

1. They are trying to protect you. All parts of us believe it is their duty to protect themselves and theoretically, by extension, you. Your body was designed to hold onto fat, so you could use it later in an emergency. Your body will not easily give up the emergency reserves. That's the rainy day savings account or the kid's college fund, not to be spent early.

2. The addiction is afraid. You chose your addiction to protect you for some reason. The addiction is like your ego, it now thinks it is you—or is better than you, that you can't survive without it. Does this sound familiar? It is the same voice as the schoolyard bully, the abuser—it is the voice of fear. Fear that they are going away. Do not taunt it or try to beat it down. You cannot beat fear that way. The only way to beat fear is to love it away. (Note: if someone else is abusing you—get help, separate yourself from that situation, do not try to literally in-person love their fear away. You only have control over you and your emotions, not anyone else's! I'm talking about loving your fear based addiction to food.)

3. Practice. You've practiced the negative thoughts and emotions for a long time. Give yourself some time to practice the positive.

I suggest you have some support while you strengthen your inner wisdom and love the old messages away. Write down your own supportive messages so that you can readily get to them. Repeat them often. Like building a physical muscle by repetition, build your mindset muscle through repetition.

As an addict, in the short-term you cannot always trust the voices, sometimes our addictions and fears masquerade as our inner wisdom.

If that is the case, how do you know if it is your inner wisdom or not?

How does the message make you feel? If you feel shame, guilt, fear, or anger, then this is not coming from your inner wisdom. Is the message in alignment with your perfect health? Do you feel empowered by the message? Are you moving towards health by following the message?

Hint: if you hear "you should" in the message that is most likely not inner wisdom. Listen for empowering "I" statements. They may be soft whispers, gentle love taps, or they may be emphatic, bold shouts from rooftops. From "I have made great progress and I feel my body needs extra rest" to "I am fed up with this nonsense. I can change. I deserve the best health."

Chapter 12: Exercising or Moving

"Movement is a medicine for creating change in a person's physical, emotional, and mental states."

~Carol Welch

The Best Exercise

> "The best exercise for weight loss is
> one that you will stick
> with...something that you enjoy."
>
> ~Laurie Tossy

A lot of people do not enjoy exercising. Especially when we are extremely overweight, exercising can be uncomfortable, sweaty, painful, and even embarrassing. I'm going to let you in on a secret about exercise—lots of people don't like to exercise, and it doesn't matter how thin they are. So, let's start by changing how we look at exercise. Instead of associating it with something distasteful, let's just look at it as moving our bodies more. That's not so hard, is it? We're not talking about working out and sweating for an hour or two. Just move your body more.

Move Your Body More

You can achieve this by walking around the block, or even walking in your house or apartment. You can park your car further away from entrances to stores. It isn't about how much you are doing right from the beginning—it is that you are committing to moving your body more. That's all.

I find boredom to be one of the biggest challenges when it comes to exercising, so mix it up. Walking is a great form of exercise, is something that most people can do, and it doesn't cost a lot of money. Just a good pair of shoes and you can be active. You can gradually add distance and difficulty. Vary where you walk so you don't get bored, even if that means some days you drive to a different place to walk. At least once a week I drive to a neighborhood that is on a hill because I love the view there. I could walk there, but then it would take too long and that walk isn't very exciting, so I get in my car and drive for 5 minutes and then walk. Other times I will drive to a pretty park or trail and walk.

I also love the "Bounce and Shake" routines that I learned from Dr. John Gray. I enjoy doing them while I repeat affirmations about my health. This is a 15 minute routine—actually he has a couple different ones. I have modified them for myself over the last couple years. I do one almost every day. They are designed for burning fat, balancing hormones, and brain chemistry. You can order the DVDs by going to http://www.RefuseToDiet.com/bounce.

Other times I might just play some music and dance. All of these ideas are inexpensive and don't require any gym membership so anyone can use them.

When To Move

> "I have to exercise in the morning before my brain figures out what I'm doing."
>
> ~Marsha Doble

I like to get my "moving" in early in the day. I have a pretty sedentary day most of the time, so this helps get my juices pumping, but I have always preferred to work out in the morning. Other people like to exercise in the afternoon because they find it helps get them over the mid-afternoon slump better than caffeine or sugar. Other people like to exercise before bed because then they fall right to sleep. That doesn't work for me because I find that exercising actually invigorates me and I am wide awake!

Experiment with when to move, but realize you are going to want to schedule it in until it becomes a habit. Don't just plan on "whenever" because that "whenever" will become "never!"

Exercising for the Obese

If you are obese or significantly overweight, you might be concerned about exercising. In addition to the typical complaints about not liking to exercise, you might be self-conscious about your appearance. Perhaps you aren't sure what is safe for you to do. Maybe you have a lot of physical pain and don't feel you physically can exercise. Or you are so out of shape you just don't know where to start.

Everyone can increase the amount they move their bodies. Again, let's get over the idea of "exercise"...we're not talking about high school PE class.

The first thing you should do, especially if you haven't exercised in a long time or if you have any health concerns, including obesity, is check with your physician or medical practitioner. The chances are really good that he or she will be fully supportive of your efforts, but ask to be sure there aren't any things that you should avoid doing that might aggravate your condition.

Studies have shown that obese women will report more aches and pains and use this as an excuse to avoid exercise. These pains are very real! Carrying excess weight is hard on your body—it stresses the joints, bones and muscles. But using the pains as a reason to not exercise keeps you in a vicious cycle.

Break that loop by taking some simple steps.

Tell yourself that you are open to being more active. This is a good basic positive affirmation! Say it out loud, many times each day.

Start your physical activity slowly so that you minimize aches and pains...and set yourself up to succeed!

Begin with 15 minutes a day. If that is too much, start with 5 minutes. Increase the amount of time until you get to 15 minutes a day.

Get support no matter what exercise method you choose. Pick someone who will help motivate you and to whom you can be mutually accountable. It doesn't have to be someone in person—it could be an online support system or someone you phone who lives across the country.

Walking is a good, basic exercise that is really portable, inexpensive and something most people can accomplish. You can walk outdoors, indoors at a mall, or even around your own home or apartment.

If walking is too difficult in the beginning, then try walking in a pool. The water will help buoy you up and makes it easier on your joints. Check in your area for a water exercise program. If you are self-conscious about getting in a swimming suit, see if they permit you to enter the water in shorts and a t-shirt. Also, see if they have a program for larger sized people. Many pools have created programs at specific hours to help their obese clients to be able to access the pool with more privacy.

Another option is to move your arms and legs while seated on a couch or even lying on your bed. This is how I had to start! When I started, my back and knees hurt so much that I couldn't move for more than about five minutes at a time—but I could move my arms and legs when I took the pressure off my feet and back. Pretend you are playing the drums and really pump your arms. Or pick your feet up and move them side to side.

You can also do isometric exercises while seated or lying down. Isometric exercises are a type of strength training. To get technical, you can either work the muscle against something that doesn't move (like a wall or the floor) which is called "overcoming isometric" or by holding the muscle in one position while it is met with resistance, called "yielding isometric." Either way isometrics work the muscles without stressing your bones and joints.

If you have had an injury or surgery, often the exercises you will be started on as part of your rehab will be isometrics.

You can do isometrics with free weights, weight machines and even elastic bands, but no fancy equipment is necessary. You can get results just by tightening you muscles and releasing and by using items that you have around the house, including your floor, kitchen counter and door frames.

Here's one quick example of an isometric exercise that will work your arms and chest:

Put your hands together in the "prayer position" with elbows high.

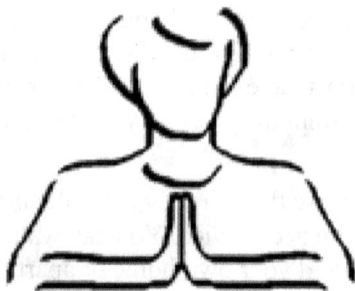

Press and hold for a count of 6 (you may have to start with a count of 3...it should be enough that you are exerting yourself but not finding it impossible to repeat.) Relax and rest for a count of 6. Repeat this three to ten times. Start with three times and work up to a longer hold count and more repetitions.

I have met a wonderful gal who is a personal trainer who has graciously provided us with some additional isometric exercises. Gena Livings has a great mindset and is in incredible shape...and can teach us a thing or two about fitness and health. Gena's isometric exercises are available in the Resources section in the back of the book.

Stick with it. Mix it up for variety. Play music or practice affirmations while you work out. If you really don't like it, try something else. There is no one right exercise for everyone. The right exercise for you is the one you will do! This is true no matter what size you are.

Find What You Can Do and Do It

The point is to find what you can do and just do it. Remember this is for your health and it doesn't take hours and hours. If you want some guidance to figure out what exercise you might prefer, ask yourself a few questions:

- Do I prefer a formal/organized program or do I prefer an informal structure? A formal program could be a class at a gym, following a DVD, or setting a time that you are going to meet friends so you walk together. Informal could be as simple as grabbing your shoes whenever you feel like it and going for a walk around the neighborhood or dancing to your favorite CD.
- Do I like to exercise with other people? Is the social aspect of exercising important to me, the camaraderie? Or do I prefer to exercise alone, either in silence or listening to my music or inspirational thoughts?
- Am I comfortable working out in public, or would I rather be in the privacy of my own home?
- Do I know enough about exercise and moving my body to be able to safely do it on my own, or do I need some education or training in this area?
- Do I stick to programs better if I make a public commitment?
- Do I like to learn new physical activities or is there something that I did in the past that I enjoyed and would like to get back to?
- Do I like loud, active environments and movements or do I prefer quiet and more stretching motions?

- How much time do I have that I will commit to exercising every day? Be sure to include the time for dressing and getting to your exercise destination.
- How much financial investment can I commit to for exercise to buy the proper attire, any memberships or instruction so I am comfortable and safe? This includes any CDs or tools you might use at home like hand weights or a good pair of shoes.
- Are there types of exercise that I just can't stand? If the answer is "all of them" then you are just going to have to start to experiment. I suggest you work on changing that mindset or you will continue to find it unpleasant—and who wants to do something unpleasant every day? Instead find something about it that you do like, even if it is when it is over!

There are going to be days when you just won't feel like exercising. It happens to me. There are mornings when my body hurts and I don't want to do it. My tip when you have days like that is to be gentle with yourself. Take some extra time for stretching, do a gentle workout and commit to only 5 minutes. Once you have done 5 minutes if you still don't feel like it then stop. It is amazing how much better I feel when I do that, even if it is just 5 minutes of exercise. I feel better because I moved my body, and also because I kept my commitment to myself.

I find that when I work out my mood gets better, so I really encourage you to just move a little bit more. Be playful with it, it doesn't have to be a serious occupation! Smile and feel love for yourself, for your body, while you move.

Examples of Exercises

Gentle on the body, and quiet: yoga, pilates, t'ai chi, walking (on land or in the water), bike riding, swimming, isometric exercises, Bounce and Shake

More active and louder: aerobics (water or land), dancing, organized sports, walking with a group, hiking, kick boxing, Wii systems

Weight bearing: walking, dancing, weight training

Do You Want a Coach?

How much exercise you do, and what type you do is going to very much depend on where you are now physically. If you decide you want to get an exercise coach, fitness instructor, or personal trainer, then I have some tips for you. For these purposes, I will use the terms interchangeably. It doesn't really matter to me what the person is called, we are talking about someone who is helping you move your body more.

Match a Coach to Your Needs and Goals

If you don't know anything about exercise, if you have been a couch potato your entire life, and you want to do something more than walking (although walking is just fine!) you should look for someone who is good at teaching you some basics in a lot of different areas. That way you can get a feel for a variety of exercises, and maybe find one or two that you particularly like.

If you know something about exercise, but it has been a while since you were active, you might want to find someone who can bring you up to speed on an activity that you used to enjoy. A lot of theories about physical activity have changed over the years and you might be surprised that what you were previously taught is no longer considered safe, or best for your muscles and bones. In addition, you have aged and your body has changed, so you might need to approach your old routine from a different perspective—a good coach can help with that so you avoid injury.

If you are obese, then look for someone who has experience working with large people. Obese people have different issues and challenges than the guy who just wants to develop his pecs or have 6 pack abs.

Has this trainer been in your shoes? In other words, did he or she ever have a weight issue more than a couple of pounds? Or were they always a natural athlete who can eat what they want and enjoy a naturally slender body?

It is not necessarily true that a person who has been fat will be the right trainer for you, but some people who have never been there just don't understand the challenges that you face, and they may not be able to relate.

Listen to your gut! A coach's job is to push you, but a good coach will inspire you, and you will feel uplifted, even though you might be tired. If you hate how you feel before, during, and after a training session then either this trainer, or this exercise, is not for you.

Look, I lost 125 pounds and I never went to a gym. I used to be a competitive swimmer, and I used to lift weights, and when I finally successfully lost weight I did it with small 15-30 minutes workouts at home, no fancy equipment (I own a lot that I've bought over the years—which are currently collecting dust in the basement!) I did my bounce and shake routines, I walked, and I focused on just moving more, being less sedentary in general.

Sometimes all the "coaching" you need is someone to remind you to move more. Someone you make a commitment to, or an appointment with. If you find you are having trouble fitting your exercise in, perhaps you need that "appointment."

You can also make a commitment by declaring it on my blog, http://www.RefuseToDiet.blogspot.com or by joining our support community at http://www.RefuseToDiet.com

Another resource is a new ebook my friend, Dr. Linda Larson has written, called *Too Busy to Exercise, Making Exercise Fit in Your Schedule*, which you can get by going to http://www.RefuseToDiet.com/easyex

> "An hour of basketball feels like 15 minutes. An hour on a treadmill feels like a weekend in traffic school."
>
> ~David Walters

The bottom line is to find a variety of ways to move your body that you can actually enjoy. The best exercise for weight loss007A is one that you will stick with...something that you enjoy.

Chapter 13: Other Tips and Tools for Success

"I have learned, that if one advances confidently in the direction of his dreams, and endeavors to live the life he has imagined, he will meet with a success unexpected in common hours."

~Henry David Thoreau

Water

While yes, there is water in the foods we eat, if you are struggling with your weight water can be one of your biggest allies. Water helps keep your body flushed and regular, and as strange as it seems, drinking lots of water helps you avoid water retention!

That being said, a lot of people are challenged by getting enough water in, so here are some tips for drinking more water.

Start the Day with Water

Start your day with a big glass, at least 8 ounces of water first thing, before your coffee, before you work out. This will help flush your system. I like my morning glass to have lemon in it. I really like how that tastes and the zing I get in the morning. Plus the lemon actually helps with metabolizing sugar. I drink 16-32 ounces in my first waking hour, but start with 8 and then you can work your way up if it feels right to you.

You do not need to sip this water—get a big amount of water in your body right away. Bill Phillips, the author of *Body for Life* likened his water drinking to a frat boy chugging beer. This is one time where you don't need to worry about being slow and savoring!

Don't Wait to Feel Thirsty

Don't wait until you feel thirsty to drink water. Keep it with you at all times, buy yourself a good water bottle that you can refill and drink all day long. Instead of having a soda, drink some water. It will help you feel hydrated and full with zero calories.

Many times we eat because we actually need water. Your body knows there is water in foods so it tells you to eat in order to get the water it needs. Head off the thirst by keeping hydrated.

I don't like tap water. I am very sensitive to the taste of the chemicals that cities put in the water to keep it clean. So I have a water filter that I use to filter out the chlorine and other additives, even though my water is perfectly safe. This allows me to drink it in the quantities that I need for my health.

If you think you don't like water, try getting an inexpensive water filter and pitcher, and see if that makes a difference.

You may not be used to drinking plain water and it really may just be a matter of getting your taste buds used to not having all the sugar and artificial sweeteners.

If filtering the water doesn't do it, then try squeezing a little lemon or lime in the water. It usually doesn't take much to do the trick. Another trick is to take a tiny splash of pure fruit juice and add it to your water. The idea is to just give your water a hint of flavor.

If you still aren't able to drink water then make some herbal tea—if you need to have it sweetened I suggest Stevia. It takes just a tiny bit to sweeten your drink; it is all natural and has no calories. I really encourage you to avoid artificial sweeteners which have been proven to actually stimulate your body to wanting more food and sugar.

I like my water at room temperature most of the time. If I have refrigerated water it is too cold and upsets my stomach. Other people prefer their water cold; it really is a matter of personal preference.

Cool weather water tip

It is easy for a lot of people to drink water when the weather is warm, but when it is cool outside sometimes drinking water is more of a challenge. Try warming up the water a little bit and splash in some fruit juice. You can also try decaffeinated green tea or herbal teas, which can give the added benefits of antioxidants. Avoid the premixed varieties in bottles as those typically are loaded with lots of sugar.

Breathe Deeply

Take deep breaths in and out. Breathing is not only essential to life it is an important part of our fitness and weight loss routines. Oxygen is part of keeping our internal fires going. Just as you can't have a campfire without it, our internal combustion works better with more oxygen. By simply getting more oxygen into our cells we can actually burn more calories—even without expending more energy!

In order to achieve the best benefit we must breathe correctly! We all breathe unconsciously...that is one of the wonders of the human body. But most of us take shallow breaths which don't gather in all the oxygen our bodies crave. And if we take a deep breath we often focus on expanding our lungs--by raising our shoulders. Check it out in the mirror. Take a deep breath. Did it look like you were shrugging?

Expand your lungs, raise your shoulders--seems logical, doesn't it? But it is wrong. To get a good, deep, fully oxygenated breath we must breathe from our diaphragm, that area above your belly button. To train yourself to breath correctly, sit down or lie on your back. Place your hand on your stomach and think about pushing your hand forward with every breath in. Practice breathing this way every day for a minute or two, five is even better. With practice breathing from your diaphragm will be second nature.

Practice your deep breathing when you first wake up and as you fall asleep. Soon you will be able to practice this breathing at your desk. Eventually you will breathe deeply, and correctly, while you are washing the dishes, walking, etc.

Get Enough Sleep

Studies show that if you short yourself on sleep you are apt to pack on the pounds. When I read that I wondered if it was the lack of sleep that caused the paunch or if it was something else. I'm no scientist, but my theory is that we tend to eat and drink more when we stay up late. Whether we are socializing, working late, or just watching television, consuming calories can help us stay awake longer, much to the detriment of our waistline. So instead of snacking, start snoozing!

Let Time Work For You

"You are investing in your health. Each small change is like a deposit to your 401(k) or IRA. Allow these small deposits to gain compounding interest."

~Laurie Tossy

Don't expect it to happen all at once. This isn't a TV show, this is your life. It is healthier for you in the long run to lose the weight slowly and keep it off, than to lose it more quickly because of lots of sudden changes that you can't, or won't, stick with.

By incorporating small changes into your life gradually, changes that are directed by your renewed connection to your inner being and self-love, you are building that strong foundation for a new you. That new you—the person who can withstand setbacks and challenges.

Think of yourself like the great Pyramids of Giza. Start by laying that first layer all the way around and then move up. Each time you complete a layer it takes fewer blocks to complete the next, until suddenly you reach the top. You have built your healthy body, one that no one can knock over because your base is so strong. This structure or way of life is beyond fad diets and gimmicks. Trust me, it will stand the test of time.

You are investing in your health. Each small change is like a deposit to your 401(k) or IRA. Allow those small deposits to gain compounding interest. This isn't a race. Time is one of your success tools...let it work for you.

Okay, I hear some of you saying, "But I want to lose weight now!" I understand, I had big goals and dreams for years about my weight, but they were so big that either:

1. I put off starting, thinking I had plenty of time
2. I started and stopped because I hit a setback or challenge

It may not be as awe inspiring to drop weight slowly—but I avoided gradual plans for years because I thought they would take too long. In the end, the slow path turned out to be significantly faster to reach the finish line. Remember the tortoise and the hare? Slow and steady wins the health race!

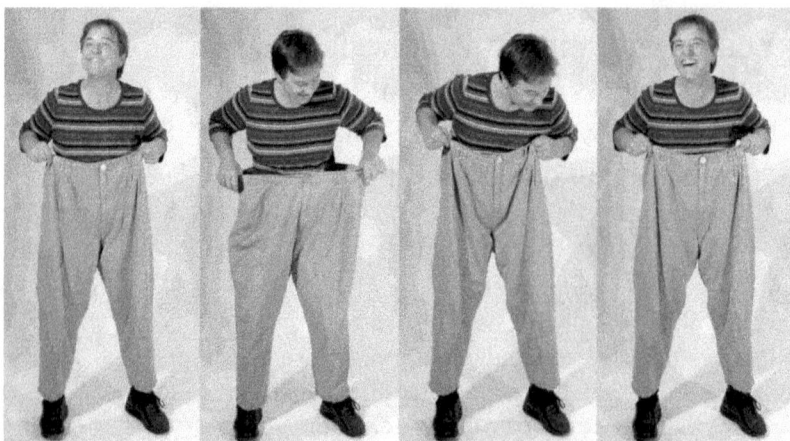

Chapter 14: Conclusion, Setting Sail

"I find the great thing in this world is
not so much where we stand, as in
what direction we are moving: To
reach the port of heaven, we must sail
sometimes with the wind and
sometimes against it, but we must
sail, and not drift, nor lie at anchor."

~Oliver Wendell Holmes

Set Off and Be Prepared to Adjust the Sails

> "I can't change the direction of the wind, but I can adjust my sails to always reach my destination."
>
> ~Jimmy Dean

Congratulations! You are setting sail on a marvelous voyage of healthy and vibrancy. Just as a sailboat must tack back and forth to get from point A to point B, you will find that from time to time you are retracing steps. That is normal and to be expected as you navigate this new course in your life.

The entire path may not be visible to you, but it doesn't need to be. On a foggy day you can see the beacon of light from the lighthouse in the distance—long before you can see the lighthouse itself...sometimes before you can even see the sea lapping at your boat. But following the light and the sound of the horn, correcting our course along the way, we can and will make it safely to our destination.

The same is true for your body image and making changes. The beacon may be your image of the perfect body and perfect health. In the fog you are experiencing today, you may not be able to see or visualize that perfection as reality. You <u>can</u> see and accept where you are now as the starting point. Then, by deciding to move towards the beacon, taking one step, one small change at a time you <u>will</u> reach that beacon...that perfection.

Three Legged Stool

Envision a three-legged stool. That is how to approach your health plan. I suggest you start with the mindset leg because that is our biggest challenge...our biggest obstacle...and where we will have the most dramatic, long-term results. Starting with mindset you will also begin to work on the food and exercise legs naturally...that is, it will flow and be a natural extension of the process.

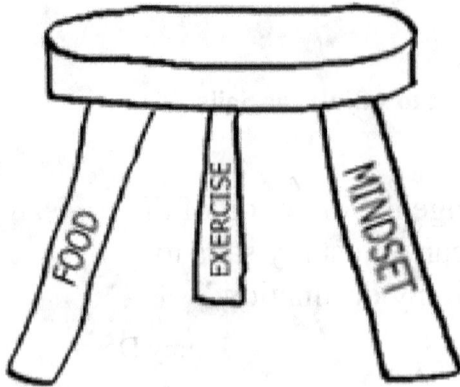

Build your health every day, leg by leg.

Every affirmation strengthens the mindset leg of your stool. Every time you move your body you are strengthening the exercise leg of your stool. And every healthy food choice you make strengthens the food leg of your stool.

By placing the focus on mindset first you will be surprised at how easily the other two legs are strengthened, as if by magic. Pretty soon you will find that you have a very sturdy and balanced stool with a crown of achievement perched on top!

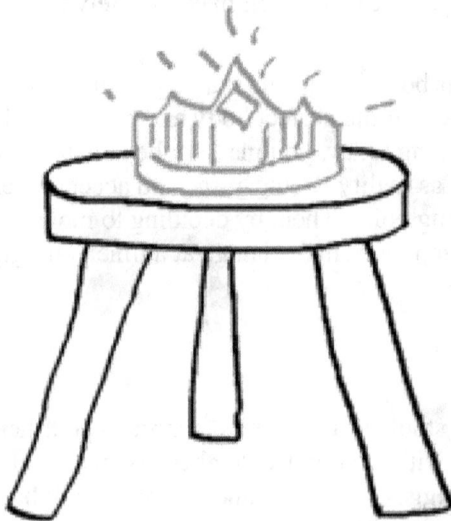

Worksheets

Lies Worksheet.

Use this to identify lies you have learned about your body, weight loss, health, dieting, etc, and how to reword them into positive affirmation.

To print out an 8.5" x 11" version, go to this website:

http://www.RefuseToDiet.com/lies

Identify the Lie	Reword it into a Positive
I crave sugar	My body desires food that fuels it
I can't seem to lose weight	I am open to the possibility that I can lose weight
My parents were fat so I will be	I have the ability to change my life and my body no matter what my parents' experience was
I can't eat my favorite foods and be slender	I can eat any foods I want and achieve and maintain my ideal weight

Who Do I Want to Be Worksheet

Use this to focus attention on what you want in life.
To print out an 8.5" x 11" version, go to this website:
http://www.RefuseToDiet.com/desires

I want: _____

I know: _____

I accept: _____

I deserve: _____

I refuse: _____

I will: _____

I _____

I _____

I _____

I _____

I _____

I _____

I _____

I _____

I _____

I _____

I _____

I _____

I _____

I _____

I _____

I _____

I _____

I _____

I _____

Options Worksheet.

Use this to identify alternatives you have to eating when feeling stressed, angry, sad, happy, etc. This is YOUR plan, options, and activities you can do other than eat-- including any tools you need to use that option so you are prepared.

To print out an 8.5" x 11" version, go to this website:

http://www.RefuseToDiet.com/options

When	I Will	Tools Needed
Example:		
When I feel stressed at work	I will go for a 5 min walk around the building	walking shoes

Affirmations Worksheet

To print out an 8.5" x 11" version, go to this website:
http://www.RefuseToDiet.com/affirmations

- I desire healthy foods.
- I love myself and take care of my body.
- I make healthy food choices easily.
- I move my body effortlessly throughout the day.
- I exercise joyfully on a regular basis.
- I am open to the possibility that I can achieve my ideal body weight.
- I have perfect health.
- My body burns fat efficiently.
- I am aware of what I eat.
- I choose foods that fuel my body.
- In every moment I love myself where I am and I have the potential to be even better.
- I love myself just the way I am.
- I love you _____ (your name), I really love you.
- I am willing to change.
- I am willing and able to change.
- My body aligns with its perfect and natural health.
- I have a healthy, slender, energetic body.
- My body craves foods that nourish it.
- My body sheds excess fat easily and effortlessly.

Reasons Worksheet

Use this worksheet to help recognize the deeper "why" behind your desire to lose weight.

To print out an 8.5" x 11" version, go to this website:

http://www.RefuseToDiet.com/reasons

Why Do I Want to Drop Weight? Note if the reason is for "A" appearance, "C" for comfort, "H" for health, or "S" for should.

The Reason

examples:

I want to be able to walk around the block without getting out of breath **H/C**

I want to be able to ride in an airplane without needing belt extensions **C**

I want to feel more attractive so I have more confidence in public **A**

My doctor says losing weight will reduce my blood pressure **S/H**

_____

_____

_____

_____

_____

_____

_____

_____

_____

Clarity Worksheet.

Use this to help identify what you DO want by first noticing what you do NOT want.

To print out an 8.5" x 11" version, go to this website:

http://www.RefuseToDiet.com/clarity

What I believe about my body, my health, my weight...

example:

What I Believe About	what I do want
I hate my huge thighs	My legs are strong and sturdy and carry me easily from place to place.

What I Believe About	what I do want

_____

_____

_____

_____

_____

_____

_____

_____

_____

Resources

Chapter 3

To print out an 8.5" x 11" <u>Weight Loss Lies</u> worksheet, go to this website:

http://www.RefuseToDiet.com/lies

Chapter 4

Michael Hebranko,
http://www.oprah.com/article/oprahshow/20090417-tows-michael-weight-loss

Chapter 5

To print out an 8.5" x 11" <u>Who Do I Want to Be</u> worksheet, go to this website:

http://www.RefuseToDiet.com/desires

Esther and Jerry Hicks, *Ask and It is Given: Learning to Manifest Your Desires*
http://www.RefuseToDiet.com/askabraham

To print out an 8.5" x 11" <u>Options to Emotional Eating</u> worksheet, go to this website:

http://www.RefuseToDiet.com/options

Affirmations:
- I desire healthy foods.
- I love myself and take care of my body.
- I make healthy food choices easily.
- I move my body effortlessly throughout the day.
- I exercise joyfully on a regular basis.

- I am open to the possibility that I can achieve my ideal body weight.

- I have perfect health.

- My body burns fat efficiently.

- I am aware of what I eat.

- I choose foods that fuel my body

- In every moment I love myself where I am and I have the potential to be even better.

To download more affirmations go to:

http://www.RefuseToDiet.com/affirmations

To print out an 8.5" x 11" <u>Reasons</u> worksheet, go to this website:

http://www.RefuseToDiet.com/reasons

To print out an 8.5" x 11" <u>Clarity Exercise</u> worksheet, go to this website:

http://www.RefuseToDiet.com/clarity

Other Affirmation Sources:
Esther and Jerry Hicks, *Ask and It Is Given: Learning to Manifest Your Desires*
http://www.RefuseToDiet.com/askabraham

Louise Hay, *You Can Heal Your Life*,
This title is both a book and a movie. The book came out first and is a real work book and very different from the movie. I have and enjoy both.
http://www.RefuseToDiet.com/hay

Other Books and Teachers Referenced in this Chapter:
Michael Losier, *Law of Attraction, The Science of Attracting More of What You Want and Less of What You Don't*
http://www.RefuseToDiet.com/losier

Eckhart Tolle, *A New Earth, Awakening to Your Life's Purpose*
http://www.RefuseToDiet.com/tolle

Claude Bristol, *TNT The Power Within You*
http://www.RefuseToDiet.com/tnt

Gay Hendricks, author and co-founder Spiritual Cinema Circle
http://www.RefuseToDiet.com/scc

Chapter 6

Dr. Linda Larson, health and wellness coach, to schedule a consultation: http://www.RefuseToDiet.com/drlinda

Chapter 9

Dr. Mehmet Oz,
http://www.oprah.com/article/health/wellnessandprevention/oz_resources_bio

Dr. Nicholas Perricone, *The Perricone Prescription*,
http://www.RefuseToDiet.com/perricone

Dr. John Gray, *The Mars Venus Wellness Solution*,
Mars/Venus Wellness Formula (shakes)
http://www.RefuseToDiet.com/gray

My Victory (shake) http://www.RefuseToDiet.com/victory

Chapter10

http://www.RefuseToDiet.com online community

Chapter 11

Dr. John Gray, retreat, http://www.RefuseToDiet.com/gray

Chapter 12

Dr. John Gray, Bounce and Shake DVDs
http://www.RefuseToDiet.com/gray

Dr. Linda Larson, health and wellness coach,
Too Busy to Exercise, Making Exercise Fit in Your Schedule
http://www.RefuseToDiet.com/drlinda

Gena Livings, personal trainer
http://www.GenaLivings.com
for Gena's isometric exercises:
http://www.RefuseToDiet.com/gena

Refuse to Diet blog: http://www.RefuseToDiet.blogspot.com

Refuse to Diet online community:
http://www.RefuseToDiet.com

Refuse to Diet Worksheets

Affirmations
http://www.RefuseToDiet.com/affirmations

Clarity Exercise
http://www.RefuseToDiet.com/clarity

Options to Emotional Eating:
http://www.RefuseToDiet.com/options

Reasons
http://www.RefuseToDiet.com/reasons

Weight Loss Lies:
http://www.RefuseToDiet.com/lies

Who Do I Want to Be:
http://www.RefuseToDiet.com/desires

Recipes

<u>Shakes</u>

I don't have a shake every day, but I frequently do, and so to have variety I have come up with some "recipes"...really they are guidelines of things you can add. Adjust the amounts to your taste.

My basic recipe
  Add ½ tbsp cacao, handful of walnuts or pine nuts
  Water as indicated on canister.

Extra chocolaty
  Add 1 tbsp cacao
  Instead of just water, use ½ water, ½ milk*

Mocha Frappe
  Add ½ tbsp cacao, 1 tbsp instant decaf coffee, ½ C ice
  Blend until slushy

Grape Tootsie Pop
  ½ C frozen mixed berries**
  Blend until slushy

Berry Vanilla Frappe
  Vanilla shake powder
  ½ C frozen mixed berries**
  Blend until thick and creamy

*use milk for ½ the volume of liquid instead of just water for a creamier shake

**Use any berries you like. Fresh berries in season are fantastic, just add ice to get the frozen texture. I have found something in blueberries makes the shakes super thick, so if you are making just a blueberry shake, use fewer berries and/or more liquid than normal.

Cookies

You can also make nutritious cookies from the Wellness Formula shake. These are not baked, but frozen, and are a healthy snack or can be used as a meal replacement. (You can try them with other shake powders, but I didn't like them when I tried making them with My Victory.)

I make up a batch using one canister of the shake mix at a time. They make 32 large cookies, each cookie equal to ½ shake.

Basic Cookie

1 canister Venus Wellness Formula shake powder (or Mars formula for men)

1 14oz jar of coconut oil, expeller pressed, unrefined (available at health or natural food stores and in some grocery stores) Melt the coconut oil. Place the jar into a pan of water on medium-low heat until melted. Let it cool slightly, but not re-solidify before adding to the other ingredients. Be sure to wipe the jar after removing it from the water, you do not want to drip water into the ingredients.

2 C Pecans, raw, organic, unsalted, use one or more to create flour. While the oil is cooling grind nuts into flour in a food processer. (A few chunks are fine.)

1/3 C cacao powder

Combine the dry ingredients in large mixing bowl and stir to mix thoroughly.

Add the oil and mix thoroughly.

Pour into a 13x9 baking dish or drop on cookie tray.

Freeze.

Variations

Sometimes You Feel Like a Nut: Add 2 C raw nuts for a nutty cookie. Use pecans, pine nuts, almonds, macadamia nuts, hazel nuts, or walnuts, whole or pieces. Garnish with a whole or half nut on top.

Poly(nesian) Wants a Cookie: Add 1 C coconut, unsweetened, ground or shredded (optional). Make sure you use the unsweetened kind; you will probably have to go to either a health food store or specialty market (many Asian grocery stores will carry this.)

Super Chocolate: Use more cacao powder and add 4 tbps cacao nibs. Cacao nibs should be unsweetened. These are hard bits and add a nice crunch.

Slender Mints: Add 5 tsp Peppermint Oil (do not use extract as it is alcohol based). I prefer these as very thin cookies.

Mix It Up: Have fun, try mixing extra chocolate and coconut, or chocolate and nuts and dust the top with coconut...

Books and Teachers Referenced Throughout the Book

Alphabetically, by last name:

Claude Bristol, *TNT The Power Within You*
http://www.RefuseToDiet.com/tnt

Dr. John Gray,
The Mars Venus Wellness Solution (book)
Bounce and Shake DVDs
Wellness Retreat
Mars/Venus Wellness Formula (shakes)
http://www.RefuseToDiet.com/gray

Mark Victor Hansen and Jack Canfield, *Chicken Soup for the Soul*
http://www.RefuseToDiet.com/soup

Louise Hay, *You Can Heal Your Life*,
The Movie and the book
http://www.RefuseToDiet.com/hay

Gay Hendricks, author and co-founder Spiritual Cinema Circle
http://www.RefuseToDiet.com/scc

Ester and Jerry Hicks, the Teachings of Abraham
Ask and It Is Given: Learning to Manifest Your Desires
http://www.RefuseToDiet.com/askabraham

Dr. Linda Larson, health and wellness coach, to schedule a
consultation: http://www.RefuseToDiet.com/drlinda

Gena Livings, personal health and fitness coach
http://www.RefuseToDiet.com/gena

Michael Losier, *Law of Attraction, The Science of Attracting
More of What You Want and Less of What You Don't*
http://www.RefuseToDiet.com/losier

Dr. Mehmet Oz
http://www.RefuseToDiet.com/oz

Dr. Nicholas Perricone, *The Perricone Prescription*,
http://www.RefuseToDiet.com/perricone

Bill Phillips, *Body for Life*
http://www.RefuseToDiet.com/phillips

Dr. Mona Lisa Schultz, medical intuitive, author, co-author of,
*Body Talk: No-Nonsense, Common-Sense, Sixth-Sense
Solutions to Create Health and Healing*
http://www.RefuseToDiet.com/drmonalisa

Eckhart Tolle, *A New Earth, Awakening to Your Life's Purpose*
http://www.RefuseToDiet.com/tolle

Brian Tracy, speaker, author
http://www.RefuseToDiet.com/tracy

9 780982 619308